Whateve. It Takes

Living with, Leaving and Surviving Psychological Abuse

Deborah Jane

Keep doing whatever it takes.

Deborah

keep going
whatever it takes.

First published 2018

Published by Forward Thinking Publishing
Text © Deborah Jane 2018

I have tried to recreate events and conversations from my memories of them. In order to maintain their anonymity, I have changed the names of individuals.

The information given in this book should not be treated as a substitute for professional medical advice; always consult a medical practitioner. Any use of information in this book is at the reader's discretion and risk. Neither the author nor the publisher can be held responsible for any loss, claim or damage arising out of the use, or misuse, of the suggestions made, the failure to take medical advice or for any material on third party websites.

A catalogue record for this book is available from the British Library.

ISBN: 978-0-9934652-5-3

Contents

Whatever it takes..1

Lights! – Looking Back at the Past and Acknowledging What Got Me Here 5

Enough is Enough, I need to Escape 6

What happened? 7

The Happiest Time of My Life.................................9

Take A Risk and Make a Change.............................20

Automatic Pilot and a Vertical Learning Curve ...26

Over-Stretched, Over-Worked and In Over-My-Head..35

Let's Keep Adding Fuel to the Fire! 41

New House,...50

New Start..50

Pay Peanuts, Get Monkeys 56

Estranged and Strange..60

Someone's Watching Over Me 66

Starting Over...72

A Christmas and New Year, Never to Forget.......76

A Glimmer of Hope 86

Fresh Start 94

Things Get Worse Before They Get Better 100

Maybe This Time? 110

History Repeating 119

Third Time Lucky 123

Act 1 – Epilogue – The Here and Now 135

Where to Get Help 137

Acknowledgements 142

This book is dedicated with immense gratitude, to my ex-husband, without whom I would not have had quite so much material. I would like to thank him for playing an integral role in getting me to where I am today and for providing me with an amazing son who is my inspiration and driving force.

Without them, I would not have adopted my mantra
'Whatever it takes'

Whatever it takes

I always wanted to write a book but didn't expect to write one about me! This book came about because too many people told me "You should write a book" based upon my experiences and I thought 'Why not?'

One day I sat down and just started to write and before I knew it I had 200 pages, which then needed to be knocked into shape. Initially, I wrote it as therapy for myself but gradually I started to write for other people, other women who might be going through something similar. Other women who felt, feel, so alone in their relationships and think that somehow it's their fault, but deep down know that it's not.

I figured that if I was going through this, then surely other people must be going through it too.

Living with, leaving and surviving a psychologically abusive relationship takes its toll. For a start it's incredibly hard to prove what is going on and you end up feeling like you're making it all up, particularly when those services and professions that you believe will help you, don't!

Picking yourself back up from a metaphorical kick in the teeth or punch in the stomach is hard work and believe me, there are times when I've re-read sections of this book just to give me the strength to keep going and to remind me of why I'm on this path.

By writing this book I hope you will feel that you are not alone. This book is my story, I hope that this will help you to find the strength to keep on going through whatever it is you're going through. Book two, Create Your Blockbuster Life, is a collation of the tips and tricks I used to keep myself going and to change my life. It will help you to make gradual changes in your life that will enable you to step out of the wings into YOUR spotlight, whatever that may be.

Bringing this book to publication has taken a number of years. Writing it took only a couple of months but fear took hold and it's only now I feel strong enough to publish. However, I have changed names throughout to protect the innocent.

Whilst writing this book I realised that I needed and wanted to learn more and thus embarked upon a BSc (Hons) Psychology with Counselling degree with the Open University. The more I have studied and learned on the subject the more I understand and the more I want to help others. My studying has had a huge influence on the direction my life is now taking and forms part of a 5-year plan that will come to fruition when I am 50.

"Whatever it takes" really is my mantra and I apply it to all areas of my life; health, fitness, finances, family and friendships, career and business.

This life really is not a rehearsal and we owe it to ourselves to create our own blockbuster and to shine in our own spotlight. You're never too old and it's never too late.

This book is one of a series. I like to think of it like a play, written in three acts and a finale or like a film trilogy. This is Act I. I've outlined the other acts so you can choose whether you wish to just read this book which tells the story and sets the scene or find out more in the next book which contains Acts II and III:

Whatever it Takes: Living with, Leaving and Surviving Psychological Abuse

Act I – Lights! - sets the scene. It tells you how this book came about, the experiences I had to go through to get to where I am today and how I believed I was destined to live permanently in the wings, lurching from one bad dramatic tragedy to the next. In short, it shines a light on my past and acknowledges its use in getting me this far and gives me the benefit of lots of lessons gleaned from lots of rehearsal time!

Book 2 - Create your Blockbuster Life: Step Out of the Wings into YOUR Spotlight

Act II – Camera! - shares the secrets of how I knew that it was time to step out of the wings into the spotlight and how I decided what it would look like when I took that step. I tell you how I created the picture of the life I wanted and how you can do the same too by using the exercises I will share in Act III to help you create the life you really want. It allows you to look through the lens to create the vision you want to see.

Act III – Action! – tells you how to take action and gives you the tools to take the action to move you out of the wings into the spotlight of your life.

Finale – Gives you a glimpse of your happy ending. The happy ending of the script you're writing that will keep you in the spotlight for as long as you desire.

Act 1, this book, is my old script. It's a book about life, it's about my life and your life, it's about getting knocked down and getting back up. It's about stepping out of the dark shadows of the wings where we've been waiting for far too long and stepping into our spotlight. It's about standing up for ourselves and our beliefs, it's about our passions and our talents. It's about discovering ourselves and finding our voice in whatever form that takes. It's about throwing off the shackles that life has bound us in, opening the curtains wide and taking centre stage. It's about remembering that life is 'Not a Rehearsal' and rediscovering our role in it. Let's step into our spotlight together, the time is now.

Lights! - Looking Back at the Past and Acknowledging What Got Me Here

"If you're going through hell, keep going"
Sir Winston Churchill

CHAPTER 2

Enough is Enough, I need to Escape

It's November 2011, the attractive, brunette, 40-year old woman sitting at her desk in her lounge has tears in her eyes and is shaking. The computer is on, its light illuminating the workspace, there's an open bottle of wine on the desk and a wine glass nearby. She's on her second glass of wine. There's also a full bottle of vodka and she's shaking as she is pushing the tablets out of their blister packs into neat piles of 10 onto the desk in front of her. There's about 5 or 6 piles there so far.

That woman is me and I remember that moment clearly.

I had reached the end of my tether, I couldn't take any more bad news or bad luck after the 3 years I'd just been through. You see, my business had become insolvent on New Year's Eve 2008 and life had become progressively worse. On that night in November 2011 I had every intention of taking my life but before the hour was out I took a decision that saved my life but would cause me to compromise every aspect of my future from that point onwards, question lots of the values and principles I held dear and simultaneously change my life for the better.

What happened?

On New Year's Eve 2008 I had been forced to make my team of staff redundant with immediate effect and no pay, my second marriage collapsed and with no-where to live my son remained with his dad. I had access to him every weekend and school holidays, but he didn't live with me. I went through personal bankruptcy and was made redundant from each of the 3 jobs I managed to get in the 18 months following my business failure. On that day in November 2011 I had just reached the end of my savings, the small amount of money I had managed to squirrel away for a rainy day. I had just been turned down for yet another job I'd applied for, I couldn't pay my rent and I had nothing left to buy Christmas presents. I was facing another Christmas wrapping up gifts that I'd managed to get from freecycle.com or charity shops. I was on the brink of bankruptcy for a second time. I had spent my last £20 on a cheap bottle of vodka, cheap wine and some pain relief tablets to bolster the stash of over-the–counter and prescription pills that were lurking in the back of a kitchen cupboard.

The future looked bleak and hopeless. I had no job, couldn't get a job, my ex-husband (my son's father) was still controlling me and using our son as a pawn, my son could see it and hated it, but I felt hopeless and helpless. I really believed the best thing I could do for everyone was to end my life. My son would never have to have divided loyalties between his constantly-warring parents, my parents would never again have to bail me out or feel disappointed by yet another failure and, I justified, whilst they might be upset initially, everyone would soon get over it and start to get on with their lives with none of the angst or problems I felt that I was continuously bringing to their doors.

It was time to take responsibility, be a big girl and do everyone a favour. It didn't take me long to drain the bottle of wine and then I opened the vodka. I took a sip to get used to the taste, I hate neat vodka, I prefer it with tonic, but I wanted this to work, there was no way I was going to dilute this magical, problem-solving elixir. The taste was sharp against my tongue, but it felt good, I knew this was going to work. I picked up the first pile of mixed pills in my left hand, I had no idea what was there altogether, but I didn't care. These unassuming white disks and ovals had a job to do. Then I reached for the vodka with my right hand.

As I tipped my head back to pour the pills into my mouth I caught sight of a photograph of my son. It was his most recent school photo. He was 6 years old and a real character. His blond hair was disheveled and his blue eyes sparkled with character and humour. He had a huge grin on his face. It was as if he was telling me in that precise moment how much he loved me and wanted me in his life more than anything in the world. Even more than chocolate spread! That look shot through me like a bullet piercing my heart. I came to my senses and realised there was no-way I could go through with it.

I put the tablets and vodka down and sobbed, letting all of my pent-up fear, loneliness, shame and despair flow through me for a good half an hour. Then exhausted, but surprisingly clear-headed, I emptied the vodka down the sink and flushed the pills down the toilet. I had the germs of a plan forming.

I couldn't believe that after all I'd been through, I was back in what felt like an even worse position than before. I felt like an abject failure, but I knew, at that moment, I had to start taking responsibility for my future. I wasn't quite sure how it was going to pan out but I knew things had to change and I was prepared to do whatever it took to create change.

How life had changed beyond recognition in just 6 short years.

CHAPTER 3

The Happiest Time
of My Life

In 2005 I had given birth to my son, Sam. He was much longed-for.

After 5 miscarriages I had given up hope of ever having a child so when I fell pregnant with him it took me up until the 8-month stage to actually believe I was really going to carry to term. Colin, my husband, had been laid off from his job on a building site and I was worried about how we would cope financially when I was on maternity leave, but being the PA to the Chairman of a privately-owned business I was assured by my boss that I had nothing to worry about and that they would look after me to ensure I could have the proper maternity leave with Sam. Unfortunately, I never had that assurance in writing and it would be one of the biggest lessons I would ever learn.

After a traumatic 39-hour labour which saw me rushed to hospital by ambulance, Sam was finally born at 1.59pm on a sunny Friday afternoon in March 2005. Due to complications and his inability to take to the breast we were kept in hospital for 3 days, where I became more and more stressed and so did he. I begged the midwives to let me go home, knowing instinctively that I'd be more relaxed at home and therefore so would Sam and, as far as I was concerned, he would then start feeding properly. I recall asking the senior midwife if they could give him some painkillers, I'd noticed what I thought was a birthmark on the back of his head at the nape of his neck and his face was quite red, as if he had high blood pressure. I firmly believed he had a headache and that this red mark on the nape of his neck was contributing to it. To say I was treated with disdain by the midwife was an understatement. I was told not to be so silly and to keep on trying to make him eat. I begged Colin to intervene, but he repeated the line I was to hear many times again "You don't know what you're doing, you've never had a baby before, leave it to the experts and just do as they tell you." By his own admission he was the "perfect parent" having fathered 3 children previously, although he had never actually lived with any one of them. I asked him to contact my parents so that they could visit me. I felt lost, scared and way out of my depth.

"Your parents have said they'll wait until you come home," was the response from Colin, who further justified it with "You're likely to be released any minute, you don't want them to drive all the way over here and find that you've gone". "But why won't they come?" I asked. I needed to see my parents and I couldn't understand why, when they'd always been there for me in the past, they seemingly didn't want to visit their new grandchild particularly when just 11 months earlier, they'd rushed to the hospital shortly after my niece was born. Even in my post-birth, new-mum haze, I knew something wasn't right. Years later I would learn that my instincts were correct.

I felt that I was getting a lot of attention from the midwives, at least that's how it seemed to me and I was grateful that I'd had a Doula present at the birth. We'd met her during an ante-natal class and as I was planning a home birth she had asked if she could volunteer her services so that she could experience what it was like to be present at a home-birth. I really didn't want anyone other than Colin and the midwife there so I was reluctant at first, but she became the compromise between Colin and I, he was adamant that I should be in the hospital from the moment anything started happening, I, on the other hand, wanted to be at home surrounded by familiar things, with my favourite music playing and scented candles burning. I hate medical intervention of any kind, I'll only take a painkiller if I'm incapacitated because of the pain I'm in and I really didn't want to be in the unfamiliar, stark surroundings of the local maternity ward. I had too many painful associations with maternity wards and even visiting it during ante-natal classes I couldn't continue the tour. Why do they insist on sending women who have miscarried or are miscarrying to the Early Pregnancy Unit which is invariably situated in the maternity unit? The pain of going through a miscarriage is bad enough, to have to go through it whilst being surrounded by women, sometimes in the next cubicle, giving birth just rubs salt into the wound. I didn't want to put any woman in that awful position and neither did I want to be aware of someone in that unfortunate position whilst I was giving birth.

The Doula visited me in the run up to the birth, she was there when I was in labour, during the birth and afterwards and she continued to visit me a couple of times a day for around a month after the birth. She was worth her weight in gold and I insisted that she was paid what she would normally charge. She and I are still in contact to this day and she has since gone on to train as a midwife and create her own blockbuster life. Any mum-to-be in her care is very, very lucky. I mentioned to the Doula that I was convinced Sam had a headache and that was probably why he wasn't feeding. Rather than pooh-pooh the idea she agreed that it was a possibility and when she returned later that day she told me that she had spoken to a cranial-osteopath about my case and that he had agreed to see a 3-day old infant. She also negotiated with the midwives that it would be better to let me go home and try to feed Sam in a more relaxed environment. I don't know how she did it but the knowledge that I was going to go home soon relaxed both Sam and me enough that he was able to suckle sufficient milk that the midwives were happy that he would not starve.

I asked my Doula why I was having so much attention from the midwives and she told me that Colin had told them he was concerned that I might suffer from post-natal depression because I'd refused to accept my pregnancy until I was 8 months and I'd never had children before and had openly said I wasn't very maternal. It's true, I wasn't maternal, but nothing had prepared me for the rush of love I felt the instant Sam was born. I told friends it was the start of the biggest love affair of my life. I'm still the same, I don't dislike children but neither do I feel compelled to spend my life as 'mum' or 'aunty' to lots of others either. In the same way I like animals, but that doesn't mean I want to live or work in a menagerie. Even after being told that by my Doula and confronting Colin with it, he managed to convince me that he was only looking after me and didn't want me to be stressed. He wanted me to be properly looked after. Something didn't ring true, but I accepted it.

Sam and I were allowed home after what felt like months but was actually only 3 days. That was 3 days too long as far as I was concerned but once we finally arrived home I started to relax properly, only to find that Colin had decorated the nursery 'as a surprise' for me. I was feeling pushed out. Whilst I was working during the latter part of my pregnancy Colin was at home and had discovered the TV sales channels. I would often come home to find that he had purchased another essential item for our unborn child. I'd had no input into the pushchair, Moses basket, changing bag or other such items that I had looked forward to researching, choosing and buying. Colin had bought them to 'help' me out and stop me 'having to worry about them' whilst I was at work. I couldn't believe how insensitive he could be to me wanting to be involved and when I questioned him about it I was told that I was ungrateful. He was trying to stop me from having too much to do whilst I was still at work and that it made him feel that he was contributing in some way because being out of work made him feel worthless. He always seemed to be able to win me around to his point of view and I gradually grew to accept that he knew best and was looking after me even though deep down I was in turmoil. I wanted to be a proper mum, I wanted to experience the excitement that went with buying my first pushchair, Moses basket, baby bath and other baby paraphernalia. I spent a lot of time feeling like I was just a vessel to carry his child rather than the mother of our child.

Gradually we fell into a routine, I was managing to breast feed our son who was feeding well after a few brief sessions of cranial osteopathy which released the trapped nerve he had. The moment I met the cranial osteopath and described what my gut instinct was telling me about Sam's inability to feed he concurred with me and after feeling Sam's head he told me that he had a trapped nerve between the two rear plates of the skull and this was causing Sam to have a headache and his tongue to loll to one side. I felt vindicated and from that point onwards, and to this day, I trust my gut instinct as far as Sam is concerned. With hindsight it's a pity I didn't trust my gut instinct in other areas of my life but more on that later.

With the bond between Sam and me growing closer through successful feeding and me loving being a new mum, my confidence was growing. I was managing to get him used to a routine and when I threw away the books that I'd been reading to help me through the first few weeks and just relied upon my instincts things seemed to get better. For a start, I wasn't constantly judging myself on how I was doing by some other person's standards and methods. I was happy and Sam was happy, but I realise now that Colin was far from happy about this bond. Every time I picked Sam up I was told to put him down "Otherwise he'll get clingy" or "You're making a rod for your own back, he won't want to go down" or "The more you cuddle him, the more he'll suffer from separation anxiety when you go back to work." I started to live for the moments when I could feed him or change him or bathe him because it felt like those were the only times I was allowed to have physical contact with Sam and be a mother.

Five weeks after giving birth I was dealt a blow, I received my payslip only to find out that the company that was going to 'look after me' had reneged on their verbal promise and I was on statutory maternity pay. Colin was out of work and my salary didn't even cover half of our mortgage, let alone pay any of our bills. What little savings we'd had had disappeared and there was no other money coming in. I begged Colin to accept one of the three jobs he had been offered but he refused, saying "They're not really me, I don't see myself doing that", "It's beneath me, I'm not doing a menial job" and "Your earning potential is far greater than mine, it makes more sense if you return to work and I'll be a house-husband".

Reluctantly I had no choice but to return to work if my family was to keep a roof over its head and food in its stomachs. In a cruel twist, I had to give my employer a month's notice that I would be returning to work earlier than planned, it meant we would go another month deeper into debt before I could do anything about getting us back on an even keel. This blow shattered my nerves and my confidence and within weeks I ended up on anti-depressants which meant I was unable to continue to feed Sam as the drugs would pass to him via me. I'd resisted the anti-depressants for as long as I could, but I was at the point where I was struggling to function properly and was constantly in tears. I needed to take them to keep me sane. My ever-helpful husband had bought me a breast pump in the run up to this moment and had insisted that I should express whatever I possibly could so that it could be frozen to enable us to feed Sam with breast milk for as long as possible. This served to make me feel even more of a failure, sitting at our breakfast bar with a pump to my breasts feeling like a cow in a milking shed. My fall into depression was assisted by a few well-timed pushes!

My first day back at work was awful. I left the house only to return home 20 minutes later as I was distraught, I'd cried from the moment I reversed off the drive and upon reaching a roundabout half way into my commute, I drove all the way around it and went home. Colin told me to "stop being silly" and to pull myself together and promised to call me at lunchtime so that I could 'talk' to our son. He'd even given me a framed photo of him to put on my desk, so I could see him every day. I don't remember much else about that day other than being told I could 'express' in the disabled toilet of the building as it was the only place I was guaranteed total privacy. My milk could be stored in the fridge in the main kitchen. I had to continue to express milk whilst waiting for my supplies to dry up and that, to me, was akin to rubbing salt in the wound. Here I was, in a situation I'd had no choice over, separated from Sam far too early whilst all the men around me were making the decisions for me without consulting me. How on earth had I ended up like this? I was starting to believe that I was incapable of making my own decisions, that the men in my life knew best, that I didn't know what I was doing and if I just did as I was told everything would be fine. Whilst these seemed like totally rational beliefs back then, I look at them now and shudder. This experience was going to have a far greater impact on the next 10 years than I could begin to imagine.

Lots of things changed that day, some of the changes were so gradual that they were almost imperceptible at first and it was only weeks, months or years down the line that I even realised things had changed.

I continued to go to work each day, my routine of reversing off the drive in tears, driving around the roundabout, returning home and being sent back out by my well-meaning, now house-husband because I had the "greater earning power" continued for a number of weeks. I did my job on auto-pilot, thankfully I'd been a PA for years and was surprisingly good at it considering I'd never ever wanted to be a PA and didn't particularly enjoy it. I wasn't qualified to do anything else, so I just accepted it, I wasn't someone who liked to challenge the status quo. I'm still someone who has very simple needs and likes and as long as my family are fed and watered and happy then I'm happy. I just accepted that having to return to work like this, with Colin unemployed and at home, whilst not my dream scenario was just one of the challenges I had to face as a new mum. After all, I reasoned, there were probably thousands of women up and down the country going through exactly the same thing as I was, and I was sure they were making a far better job of just getting on with it. I told myself that I had to stop acting like a princess and put up and shut up. At least I still had a job, I had a husband, a baby, a nice house and a nice car. I've always been an optimist and able to see something good in just about every situation but reading that reasoning as I've written it I see that I was quite the Pollyanna. I took a deep breath, set my jaw, adopted a stiff upper lip, and got on with it as best I could. I'd been brought up to be a good girl and to do as I was told in a family that firmly believed in the stiff upper lip, so that's just what I did.

It wasn't long before I was exhausted. I was emotionally drained each day, busy in work and then coming home to cook dinner, do the housework and collapse in a heap on the sofa for an hour before going to bed. Each day, in order to 'help' me, Colin would get up with our son before I left for work and undertake the breakfast routine so that I could 'get ready for work in peace', I'd have my lunchtime telephone call with our son which involved me calling his name and talking to him and Colin describing his reactions to me.

Occasionally if I was lucky I'd hear him (Sam) gurgling down the phone, this would keep me going until the evening.

I would arrive home from work at around 6pm to find that Colin had 'helpfully' undertaken the bath time routine and I would be allowed to settle Sam to bed somewhere between 6.30pm and 7pm. Invariably I'd end up ousted from this as my presence was making Sam too excitable at bedtime. The reality quickly became me seeing Sam briefly before I left for work each morning and then kissing him goodnight when I arrived home from work. Again, I told myself that this was what most fathers went through each day and that the only difference with us is that mum was the breadwinner and provider and dad was responsible for the childcare.

I hated it with every fibre of my body but that was the way it had to be. Someone had to take responsibility for providing for my family and Colin had made it quite clear that he wasn't prepared to do that! In fact, the only thing Colin was prepared to do was be 100% focused on our son, to the detriment of everything else. On top of working full time I was doing the shopping, cooking and cleaning then being grateful for being allowed to be a proper mum at the weekends. All this meant, of course, is that I still had to do everything but with Sam in tow. My favourite times were our Saturday mornings when I walked him in his pushchair to the local butcher and greengrocer. I loved putting him into the baby seat in the trolley and pushing him around Tesco. I felt like a proper mum when strangers would stop and coo over him. My heart would swell with love and pride and for a few brief moments I would forget that my reality was as far removed from everything I had ever imagined it would be. I clung on to those moments.

Strangely, whilst going through this crisis I was having some flashes of lucidity and the germ of a seed of an idea was beginning to grow in my mind. I have always been interested in ways of bettering myself. Despite not going to university I had a thirst for knowledge and if I wanted to learn about something I would go and buy books or a magazine on the subject matter I was interested in and devour them until my questions were answered and my thirst sated. I'd started to hear some interesting things about Virtual Assistants in the USA; they appeared to be PAs who had given up their full-time job to work for themselves from home whilst using the power of the internet to undertake secretarial services for clients all over the world. This sounded quite space-age and 'out there' to me but it also intrigued me. What if I could work from home? What if I could learn to use the internet in the same way as they did? What if I could do something similar?

From a position of desperation, I had possibly found a solution. A really scary, almost unthinkable solution but a possibility nonetheless. But could I dare to dream it was possible? It was the only thing I could possibly do that would enable me to be at home with Sam and be the mother I wanted to be. The prospect made me almost sick with excitement. The potential reality of it terrified me and I tried to push it to the back of my mind, but this seed was growing stronger and stronger and would not be quietened no matter how hard I tried.

I started to spend my evenings using my computer to do some research instead of slumping onto the sofa before bedtime. I wasn't really sure what my plan was, but I could develop that when I knew a bit more about these virtual assistants and how it worked. I have to say that these were the days long before the 'cloud' and well before Facebook and Twitter had come into existence. We were using dial-up at home and most businesses were still using dial-up too. I had a lot of research and learning to do before I could even dare to dream but how could I possibly accept or reject the dream before I had any cold hard facts?

With more than a little trepidation I shared my burgeoning idea with Colin, he was incredibly supportive and in just a few short weeks we had a far better idea of what we would need to do.

My idea had suddenly been hijacked by Colin, he could see that this was a great way of earning more money than I currently earned and it meant I would be at home with him and could see our son. Of course, I'd have to ensure I worked in a home-office and be disciplined about the time I spent with our son, we didn't, he chided me, want our son to be thrown from his routine now that he was happy and settled.

I/we started to develop a list of the services we/I would be able to offer from home. To be honest whilst it was fun undertaking this exercise I really didn't believe it would be any more than that, a research exercise which would ultimately tell us that to do this from home would be far too costly and far too difficult to ever get off the ground in the UK. And that was the conclusion we had more or less arrived at.

CHAPTER 4

Take A Risk and Make a Change

One Thursday afternoon in September 2005 I arrived home from work early and Colin was surprised to see me. I had been back at work for just around 3 months and whilst I'd been teasing myself with this virtual assistant idea that's all it was, a distraction that stopped me from bursting into tears all the time, I was still on anti-depressants and still quite fragile. As I walked through the door I answered Colin's quizzical expression with.

"I've quit".

"What do you mean you've quit? You've resigned?"

"No, I mean I've quit with immediate effect."

"You can't do that, how are we going to live, how are we going to pay the bills?"

"I don't know, but I'm not going back, I'll take in typing and earn money doing that virtual assistant thing, it can't be that difficult. I'll be a freelance PA."

That afternoon the Chairman who I was a PA to had been in a foul mood, he'd called his board into an unplanned meeting to discuss something with them. I'd put the required papers on his desk earlier that day. He had been working with the papers throughout the day and put them down somewhere safe as was his wont. He'd stormed into his office from the board room, had a rummage around, couldn't find the papers, called me to search for them and when I'd looked and been unable to find them had yelled at me, for all of the board to hear "I'm not happy."

Something inside me just snapped.

Our relationship had never been the same since I returned to work, he didn't like no longer being my top priority and I resented the way he had misled me. I knew that I wouldn't be working there until I retired which is what I'd originally planned but I didn't expect to be leaving quite so soon either.

"Right" I thought as I watched him storm back into the board room and slam the door.

With a calmness and presence of mind that I've rarely had when making a massive decision, I logged off from my computer, collected all of my personal effects and left my office, locking the door behind me. I put my bag on the floor and entered the HR Director's office. She and I had become firm friends through our time working together, we were the only women in the company who had the ears of the board and the privilege of sitting around the board table and between us we created a solidarity, somehow managing to strike the balance of stroking the egos of the men sat around the table whilst challenging some of their thoughts and ideas and gaining their respect. She had been a massive support to me when I returned to work and I was grateful for her calm and measured manner on more than a number of occasions.

She looked up from her desk as I entered and said to her "The Chairman says he's not happy so I'm giving him something to be unhappy about. Here's my keys, I quit" I could see my words going around her mind and her trying to figure out what exactly I had said, but before she could say a word I turned and left. I was just driving out of the car park when my mobile phone rang.

"Am I right in thinking you've just resigned?"

"No, I've quit with immediate effect."

"Don't be hasty, take the weekend, come back in on Monday and we'll talk about it."

"I don't need until Monday, I'm not coming back"

"Well, I'll call you on Monday to see how you are."

And that was it. In less time than it takes me to choose what to eat from a restaurant menu I had made a life-changing decision without asking for anyone else's advice or guidance. Colin was just going to have to deal with it.

That evening Colin told me I had no choice but to become a freelance PA. "You'll have to take in typing and work out how to offer everything else." By now remorse had set in as I realised what I had done, and I had no idea how I was going to turn our dreams of a few weeks into a reality. I was terrified, and my response was not what he wanted to hear "No, you're going to have to take one of the jobs you've been offered." I could almost hear his excuses before he opened his mouth; "They're not for me. I wouldn't be able to stick at it. Your earning power is far greater than mine. You like working. You love the cut and thrust of business. You're not at all maternal, you won't be happy being a stay-at-home mum. You'll get bored being at home all day, you're used to being at work..." and so they rolled on.

I knew that asking him to take a job was futile. In my gut I recognised that once again, I'd ended up with a husband who had promised me the earth until he had me as his wife, then the goal posts were shifted and I was expected to be the provider. It had happened with my first husband and here it was happening with my second. I felt sick but knew that the only way I could keep a roof over Sam's head and ensure he was well fed and looked after was by doing 'whatever it takes' to earn some money.

After a sleepless night, I awoke the following morning and thoroughly enjoyed the novelty of being able to give Sam his breakfast. I could have done without Colin wittering on about how I was doing it wrong and how Sam was fractious because he wasn't used to mummy feeding him and how I was ruining Sam's daily routine and wasn't it about time I got on the phone to try to get a job! I was 'wasting' valuable time with Sam which should have been spent working or trying to get work. This was to become a mantra I would hear often over the following months and years.

Shortly, I picked up the telephone and started calling the one or two people I knew who might be able to offer me some work or know someone who could. I started with the employer I'd worked for immediately before going to work for the Chairman I'd just walked out on. He was the UK Managing Director of a global engineering company. Although I hadn't realised it then, this was my first foray into business networking and word-of-mouth referrals. I told him my predicament and he suggested we meet for coffee a day or two later.

Prior to meeting David, my former employer, for coffee I revised the business plans I had been half-heartedly creating with Colin during my maternity leave. The more I read them the more I began to realise that I might just have the beginnings of a business and armed with little more than an idea, lots of hope and an increasing sense of desperation I went to meet the person who would become not just my very first client, but also my informal business mentor.

I knew that David was planning his retirement, I'd started working for him as his PA some 5 years earlier and even at that stage he was planning to retire 'sometime in the next 2 years'. Naturally that 2 years had been extended to a little longer, but he was now in the first throes of retirement by working on a consultancy basis for the company we had both worked for. Having been an engineer all his life and swiftly rising to the ranks of senior manager and then Director, he had never had to use a computer himself. His career had started when everything was typed up by secretaries, PAs and typing pools and he had then had a PA when systems transferred from manual to electronic.

Despite only having worked for him for 2 years I had become well-used to hearing anguished exclamations coming from his office when his computer crashed or his emails 'disappeared'. He was used to having his life organised for him and having to focus on just the important aspects of the job he was paid to do. He was good at his job and highly respected, he'd even served as an expert witness on skyscraper buildings following the atrocities of 9/11, both of us watching the BBC news stream on an intermittent internet connection from my office and realising that the entire Board of this massive organisation, excluding him, were somewhere within the vicinity of the twin towers that morning. It's fair to say that was a pretty tough day at the office but it cemented our relationship as a team.

I was looking forward to catching up with him, running my idea past him and seeing if he had any suggestions.

Although I was looking forward to catching up with the person who was my favourite boss, I was also nervous. He didn't suffer fools gladly and if he thought my idea was ludicrous or a no-go he would tell me gently but in no uncertain terms.

I quickly brought him up to date with the events of recent weeks and then after answering some well-meant questions about my welfare and what Colin was proposing to do to help alleviate the situation, I tentatively told him about my idea.

I wanted to offer PA services to semi-retired Executives and non-exec directors who had been used to having their own PA but now found themselves having to do all of their admin themselves. My idea was to buy a server so that clients could dial-in to their own space on the server and pick up any work I had done for them or even access emails and their online calendars. Outlook has always had that functionality and having worked in a number of global organisations. I knew that it could be harnessed as an effective business tool whilst on the go.

I had no idea quite how I was going to get the server but for now that didn't matter, what mattered was that I could sell the bigger picture whilst delivering most of it in bite-sized chunks.

David was impressed and intrigued, enough to volunteer himself as my first client. I hadn't been expecting that and when he asked me what my rate was I didn't have a clue. We agreed upon £25 an hour and he sent me away with a list of things I needed to get in place in my business before we actually started to work together again. The list read something like this:

1. Create a financial forecast

2. Find a solicitor to write a client contract

3. Find an accountant

4. Write a business plan to present to a bank

5. Think about and create a marketing strategy

6. Think about my plans for growth

I had a lot of work to be getting on with!

CHAPTER 5

Automatic Pilot and a Vertical Learning Curve

I think I was a bit shell-shocked following that meeting and it had nothing to do with the two cups of black Americano I had drunk. I'm hopeless with coffee, I'm not a huge fan of it and anything more than one cup of weak instant coffee in a day has me bouncing off the ceiling from the impact of the caffeine. I wasn't sure if I was feeling sick and light-headed because of that, or if it was because "I think I've just got a client" as I said to Colin on the brief telephone call before I drove home. Perhaps it was because of the list of things David had told me to put into place which terrified me! Whilst I knew from my previous job that a major international business needed all of these things, did a work-from-home freelance PA really need to create a marketing strategy? Was I really going to earn enough to require an accountant? Why did I want to have a formal contract when

I was only planning on working a couple of hours per month for each client?

Although I understood how businesses worked and, Colin was right, I really did love the cut and thrust of big business, I was ridiculously naïve in thinking that what applied to big business didn't apply to small businesses. At the very core of all businesses they are the same and it's their processes, procedures, contracts and trusted advisors and professionals that keep them going.

My learning curve became vertical. Before I knew it, I was meeting the bank to set up a bank account and joining the FSB (Federation for Small Businesses). The small business advisor at the bank invited me to an all-day business networking event and told me to ensure I had plenty of business cards. I had no idea what a networking event was and even less of an idea of what was expected of me but not to be deterred I created some very basic home-made business cards and off I went. I was proud of my cards, I had a business name and logo (courtesy of WordArt) and my name and the words Managing Director appeared below the logo. On the back were the logos of my professional organisation, IQPS (the now-defunct Institute of Qualified Private Secretaries) and the FSB. I felt like I had arrived!

I will never forget that business event.

It taught me many, many lessons about starting a business and many more about myself. It was co-hosted by my bank and a man called Robert Craven of The Director's Centre, neither of whom I'd ever heard of. I entered the room full of suits feeling sick to my stomach. Whilst I love being on a stage and performing to an audience I have never been good at small talk and was dreading having to make polite conversation with lots of business people who obviously knew far more about business than I did. They were obviously successful, and I was just a wannabe trying to convince them that I was a business person.

However, I managed to quell my nerves and listened to the man, Robert Craven, separating the small, one-man-band businesses from those with 6 employees or more. Whilst I was technically a one-man-band, I wasn't going to let anyone else know that this was my very first event. I talked about my office (our spare bedroom) and my team (Colin, son, parents and sister – all of whom I knew were willing me to succeed in this crazy, scary venture). It didn't matter to me that my office and team didn't exist, in my mind I'd created a back-story for the character that was the Managing Director of Virtual PA Ltd.

Two things happened at that event that made me more determined than ever that I would not be a failure.

1.   Robert Craven asked us all to place one of our business cards on a table at the back of the room. Throughout the course of the event he would take some time to look at them and offer feedback on how effective they were. Naturally I placed my card on the table, feedback was all important, I couldn't fail at this venture.

2.   During one of the seminars Robert Craven asked for volunteers. Even before I knew what he was asking for volunteers for, I felt my right arm fly up past my ear and wave my hand in the air. It was a completely subconscious response and one I can only put down to nerves and desperation. I was selected as one of the volunteers!

The room had been set up with approximately 20 tables of 10 people per table. I noticed that there was one volunteer per table. We were then asked to stand on top of the table whist we listened to instructions of what we would be required to do. At this point I wasn't too worried, I was used to performing to audiences and I was good at taking direction, this would be OK. But then he added, "You have 90 seconds to deliver your elevator pitch to the room." If my jaw didn't actually drop to the floor it certainly felt like it had!

What the heck was an elevator pitch?

I listened to two other volunteers before it was my go. They seemed to be describing quite succinctly what their businesses were or did. They made perfect sense to me and I felt confident, if a little nervous, that I could describe my freelance PA business quite cohesively in the allotted time. This was little more than ad-libbing on stage, or so I thought. Knowing that what I was offering was practically unheard of in the UK at the time I decided that it was best to educate the audience whilst I had their attention and they were open to it. I opened my mouth and started to describe how clients would dial into a server to get their work in just the same way as they had been used to in their working lives. I went into intricate detail about how it would work and when 3-minutes had elapsed Mr Craven told me to stop. He then proceeded to use my elevator pitch as an example of how not to make an elevator pitch. I was mortified, here I was, on top of a table pitching my business to a room full of strangers and as far as I was concerned this man was very publicly shooting me down in flames. I've since learned that he was actually doing me and all those other business owners a big favour, he continued to teach us how to put an elevator pitch together and hone it so that it was succinct and memorable.

Whilst I wanted the ground to open up and swallow me whole, at that moment I sat back down thinking "Well, I might have got the elevator pitch wrong but at least 250 people now know I exist." That was my baptism of fire into getting my business name (and my name) out there with no marketing budget. I was soon to get me, and the business, noticed again by the people in the room.

My very public humiliation was only just starting!

Shortly after the elevator pitch debacle, we revisited the business cards on the table at the back of the room. He stopped at each card that had been placed by a small business owner and started to critique it. Wrong colour, wrong font, wrong pitch, too much white space, not enough white space, it doesn't say what you do, where are you based? Where's the fax number? Yes, those were the days when businesses still had faxes. We hadn't quite progressed to scanning and emailing documents! Where's your website address? Email address? The list was endless, and he hadn't got to my card yet. Having initially felt quite proud with what I'd managed to create at short notice with no budget I was starting to feel quite ill. He was getting closer to my card, three cards away, two cards, one card "Whose is this? Where's Deborah-Jane?" he asked waving my card in the air and reading my name from it.

I waved my hand in the air, feeling for the second time that day, that I wanted the ground to swallow me whole. I stepped forward as he addressed me and everyone else stepped back so that they could all get a good look.

"This is obviously home-made; it shows you're not at all serious about your business, that it's a life-style business and the use of these logos on the back just confirm that you're a small business." My heart sank, here I was again putting myself in a position of public humiliation when all I was trying to do was support my family. It took all I had not to burst into tears and flee from the room. I felt hopeless, useless and stupid, what would Colin say? What would Sam (who couldn't yet speak) say? What a laughing stock I had become! I had so much negative self-talk going on in my head that I almost didn't hear the few words of praise from him following my response to this very simple question:

"How long have you been in business Deborah-Jane?"

"Umm, about 10-days." was my mumbled response, eyes cast downwards, refusing to make eye-contact, and trying to work out my escape route. "How many of you here have been in business for less than 6 months?" asked Robert to the assembled 250 bystanders of this public shaming. Not a single hand went up. Just as I was about to garble something of not knowing this was event was only for established businesses and that my bank manager had invited me.

Robert addressed the whole room, "There are 250 of you here representing at least 200 different businesses. You have all had the same opportunities presented to you today and Deborah-Jane is one of only a handful of you who took the opportunity to pitch their business to the entire room. Some of you haven't even put a business card on this table. So whilst Deborah-Jane may not have got it right, there are now 250 people who know her and her business who didn't know about it yesterday. How many people have you pitched your business to in the past 10 days? Two hundred and fifty?"

I was confused. Had I done something right or wrong? Was he insulting me or complimenting me? It took me a long time to realise that he hadn't shot me down in flames as I'd felt he was doing, but he had in fact held me up as an example to be applauded for taking the risk. However, going home that day, I felt like an abject failure. If this was what building a business was all about I needed to learn a lot more before I ventured out to a networking event again!

Needless to say, I learned quickly. I said my learning curve was vertical, it wasn't so much a curve as a straight line. I had a sense of urgency in all that I did, and I became a sponge, soaking up as much business advice as I could possibly take in. I revised my business card, learned what an elevator pitch was and created several and I attended as many networking events as it was possible to attend. Slowly but surely clients started to sign up to my new legal contract that had been drawn up at great expense by a solicitor.

Within three months of that first event I was struggling to keep on top of work by myself and once again Colin had the 'perfect' answer. Recognising that networking was bringing my clients in and it was clients who were paying our bills and also recognising that if I couldn't take on any more clients then we couldn't increase our household income (without him getting a job – I added that bit, he never suggested that!), then it was perfectly clear to him that he should assist me in the business when our son was asleep. I could go out networking, grow the business, sign up more clients and he could stay at home, be a house-husband whilst answering the phone, responding to emails, and generally ensuring that not a single opportunity to grow the business was missed.

I argued that growing the business wasn't the issue, it was getting the work done that was the problem and he responded that whilst 'we' were on a roll, it was vital that I was out and about as the face of the business, I could come home and put our son to bed then get client work done in the evenings. I argued that I needed some rest time, but he countered that by telling me that all entrepreneurs put in ridiculous hours during the early days of building their business but that within a year or two I'd be able to pull back and spend time as a family. We'd have a team of staff whom we could trust to run our business.

I recall thinking to myself "It's not *our* business, it's *mine*," but thought nothing more of it. I was the sole shareholder and director, he was listed as the company secretary for legal reasons but other than that he had no entitlement to the business (back then you had to have a Director and Secretary to set up a Limited company). He reasoned with me that it wouldn't be too long before I could take on a proper secretarial assistant and for the short-term, whilst 'we' built up some money, this would be the best way forward. So I started networking from 6am most mornings, occasionally returning home during the middle of the day to undertake an hour or two of work before going back out again to a networking event. If the event went on into the evening, I started delivering client work when I arrived home. It quickly became the norm for me to start working at 10 p.m, finish at 2 a.m and then be up again at 5.30 a.m for another 6 a.m or 6.30 a.m breakfast network. I got used to surviving on a diet of cooked breakfasts, black coffee by day and white wine by night. Before too long I was drinking a full bottle of wine most evenings to send me to sleep, then getting up, showering, and heading out of the door fuelled by coffee and 3 or 4 hours of sleep.

Logically I knew that this was not a routine I could continue for very long, but each time I complained to Colin or asked for help he would somehow soothe me and tell me it wouldn't be for long and it would all be worth it in the end. I've always been a big picture thinker, preferring to know what the small steps are working towards for them to feel of value. As soon as I know the big picture, I'll generally do *whatever it takes* to ensure I achieve it.

Another three months passed, and I was feeling ill. Colin, by now, had decided he needed to take over the strategic and operational direction of the business to free me up to focus on client delivery and PR and marketing as he classed networking. "Besides" he reminded me, "You like networking and you're the face of the business now, no-one can do it as well as you can, you'll just need to manage your time more effectively." Although I agreed with him, I put my foot down and insisted on getting some help. He interpreted this as me not knowing what I was doing and hired an extremely expensive business coach.

I didn't need a coach, I needed someone to help alleviate my workload. I needed Colin to step up, be a man and actually give me some proper help, either in the house or in the business.

I couldn't continue to do it all whilst he convinced himself, me and many other people that he was in fact my knight in shining armour and holding the fort at home and in the office whilst I was off gallivanting at networking jollies and 'choosing' only to deliver client work in the evenings or early hours of the mornings.

I felt trapped, I knew that if I didn't carry on as we were there would be no income, no food on the table and eventually no roof over our head. I pleaded with Colin to reconsider some of the jobs that he had been offered, but he refused. He decided that he had been at home too long and self-employed for too long to be able to work for anyone else. I was constantly reminded of my father's words during his speech at our wedding, "irresistible force meets immovable object." Both Colin and I were stubborn but in different ways, I had a relentless determination to achieve my goals, his stubbornness was about getting his own way. Whilst I was always prepared to compromise as long as I didn't lose sight of where I wanted to be, he was all about getting things done his way without compromise. Compromise was for the weak and anyone not agreeing with him on anything was wrong, it was unacceptable that they could possibly have a different opinion to him, they were just wrong!

If someone told him the sky was blue and provided him with evidence that it was blue, he would insist it was red if that is what he genuinely thought. There would be no room for discussion, consideration or compromise. If the other person would not agree with him they were wrong. The conversation would be ended and he would walk away, hang up the telephone or decide that he could never talk to, see or work with that person again because they didn't have a clue what they were talking about. He was a master of getting people to agree with him most of the time and he was a master at convincing people that he was helping them out, that he was putting his needs last to ensure that they got what they needed.

Hindsight is a wonderful tool and going back over my story whilst writing this book, I can see the patterns emerging and the signposts clearly directing the path that my life was becoming destined to take for the next few years. However, at that point in time, I was so stuck in what the reality of the situation was, I really couldn't see what was clearly happening in front of my face.

CHAPTER 6

Over-Stretched, Over-Worked and In Over-My-Head

The business coach came on board. He was a very nice man and we got on well despite me constantly telling him that I wasn't in a position to hire a coach and at this stage in the business what I needed was some hands-on help, not a coach. Both he and Colin constantly rolled out the analogy that in order to become a professional athlete, sports people had coaches to help them improve and so businesses needed coaches to enable them to compete. I had no problem with understanding the value of a coach, but I also knew I couldn't afford one. I was just about bringing in enough to cover our household costs and pay for the few hours a week of junior admin support I was hoping for, I couldn't afford the £1,000 plus per month that a business coach would cost.

Undeterred and deaf to my protestations, Colin ploughed on with his plans for my business. A business that he readily admitted he was uncomfortable delivering to my target clients as he couldn't relate to them and didn't understand their needs. When he had been in work he'd been a games machine designer and then an electrician on a building site, hardly the credentials required to help him deliver the requirements of executives and non-executive directors. I was growing more and more resentful of my business but knew that if we were to keep our house, food on the table and petrol in our cars that I needed to go along with it. We needed to be united and I allowed myself to be lead along a route I didn't want. After all, I was a good actor and it was easier to pretend that I was playing a part and researching a role than it was to face the reality unfolding in front of me. If I faced up to what was really happening I would have had to admit that my marriage was a mess, my business was struggling, and I really wasn't as strong and confident as I appeared. There was too much at stake for me to face reality. I figured that I'd created this situation, so I had to make the best of it and buy myself some time to work out how to change it!

It only took about 3 sessions before the business coach and Colin decided that we needed to prepare for exponential growth. It was, they decided, blatantly obvious that the business would grow, after all it had already exceeded my expectations and I was blasting every growth objective I set myself. That wasn't difficult, I needed something to aim for, I always had. It kept me focused and driven. More to the point, it kept my mind off the reality of what was going on in my marriage. As Shakespeare said, "All the world's a stage." I'm not sure he meant for me to take it quite so literally.

As a child I'd wanted to be a nurse and I learned all I could about nursing. I even joined the St John Ambulance Brigade at the age of 8, rapidly rising through the ranks of Cadet Corporal, Cadet Sergeant, Cadet Leader to Grand Prior's Cadet; the highest award a cadet could achieve. Realising that looking after people also meant clearing up excrement and vomit, I knew at the young age of 12 that I really couldn't do that for life, so I changed my focus to acting. I discovered drama when I went to comprehensive school having only previously appeared in primary school nativity plays and Christmas productions but drama in 'comp' was different. I felt at home and learned with some irony that the only place I really felt alive and like 'me' was on a stage, when I was being someone else.

Although I didn't know it then, that feeling was going to be with me for a very long time. On a stage I felt free, even if I was pretending to be someone else. I got a sense of freedom from pretending that I never felt when I was just being myself. I always felt that 'me' wasn't quite good enough. My goal swiftly changed to that of getting my equity card and at the age of 14 I joined a local amateur drama group to gain valuable performance experience with my eye firmly on my end goal.

So, whilst I was surprised that the Business Coach happily talked about growth with Colin and me, and I erred on the side of caution, not wanting to over commit ourselves, or rather me, financially or in terms of ability to deliver the work, I quickly found myself moving out of the home office to a small office in a local business centre. This was the last thing I wanted. I was deeply uncomfortable with taking on the additional overhead and managed to negotiate that if we were growing it was time to take on staff. The business was only just 6 months old. I was now committed far more than I ever wanted to be and worse still I also had someone else dependent upon me making sales so that she could pay her bills. I hated the burden and the responsibility. Whilst I was happy to take responsibility for myself and my actions, I hated being responsible for what was in reality someone else's lifestyle.

I was aware that I was becoming more and more withdrawn into myself and that every time I went out to network or promote the business I was putting on an act. Colin didn't notice, the more I said that I couldn't cope or needed a break the more he insisted that I loved it really and just needed to get out networking more. Before long I had taken on more staff and ultimately ended up with a team of 6 PAs all working under Colin's watchful gaze whilst I went out and brought home the bacon for all of them.

I was leaving the house at 6am each morning, attending a networking event, arriving at the office mid-morning, occasionally attending a networking lunch, returning to the office mid-afternoon, popping home to kiss Sam goodnight, heading off to yet another networking event, arriving home after 10pm, using the home office to undertake client work or some other paperwork that I was required to do for the business before collapsing into bed in the early hours only to repeat it all again the next day.

Colin by this time had decided that as he was now vital to the smooth running of the business our son should go into a nursery.

He had been attending a childminder for a few days each week but as Colin decided that the registered, well known, highly recommended and respected childminder, whom I had chosen because she was also a good friend of mine and had the same values and principles as me, was no longer at the right standard (in other words, she had ventured her opinion on something regarding our son and Colin didn't agree with her so decided she was wrong and didn't know what she was doing).

Our son therefore had to go into a full time registered nursery. The cost was almost double what I was already paying, and I was feeling even more crippled by the financial burden being placed upon me.

I was spending less and less time with Sam, more and more time working and generally hating the situation I'd ended up in. Whenever I considered giving it all up and finding a job Colin would remind me of how many people depended upon me to bring in the business so that they could pay their bills.

Neither of us were taking a salary from the business, but in order to stop him feeling emasculated he had asked me to transfer payment of the child benefit and child tax credits to him.

Colin justified that he felt emasculated working for his wife in a female dominated industry and not earning a salary made him feel even worse. He blamed this for his lack of drive and motivation and assured me that as soon as we were both taking a salary the child benefit and tax credits would be returned to me as the mother and he would feel much happier about being in my shadow. To avoid further arguments, I transferred the payments to him. That was a decision that would cost me dearly in years to come.

The business continued to grow, the costs continued to spiral, and our team rapidly grew. Our total salary bill each month was in excess of £10,000 before I paid any other bills. Whilst on the one hand I felt quite proud and secretly surprised at my ability to bring in that sort of revenue, our spiraling costs terrified me. Colin, knowing my concerns seemed at the same time to be oblivious to them.

Before I knew it we had brand new office furniture and an all singing, all dancing website. I hated the website. It was taking far too much of my time as I was having to proof read the text the copywriter had written to ensure it was accurate. Unsurprisingly, it wasn't me who had chosen to update the website or hire a copywriter. I had however, agreed to the new office furniture. The furniture we inherited in our office was shabby, worn and tired and not really fit for purpose.

I knew that it was important that we presented a smart and efficient image to any clients who might visit us and I wanted some decent storage for our files. I needed to run an efficient office that much I was certain of. 'Tidy desk, tidy mind' was my mantra and whilst, like anyone, I would often have papers strewn over my desk whilst I was working, I also insisted upon a place for everything and everything in its place. Each evening before I left the office, my desk would be cleared. I never left work half completed, and I would write my to-do list in readiness for the next day so I knew exactly what was on the schedule. I also pencilled in time to allow for any unexpected work or meetings.

The office was OK.

He volunteered and got agreement from the landlord, to paint the office in our corporate colours, which made it look and feel 100 times better. The external elevation wasn't great but once inside it did at least seem to live up to the image I wanted to project of the brand. Bizarrely, whilst all this was going on, I was becoming more and more unhappy. I realised why I was unhappy. Superficially the business was doing well and for all his faults Colin was at least focused on making it work, albeit to his specifications, but it was better than him not being supportive. I, however, was losing sight of the reason I'd started the business in the first place. For me it had been about being a mum whilst maintaining some identity of my own. All I wanted was to be mummy to Sam. It's all I've wanted since he was born. I had started the business to bring in an income whilst allowing me extra time to be with him. I was bringing in more than enough income, but it wasn't allowing me the time that I craved with Sam.

I felt that my life and my mind was spiralling out of control and I had no idea how to change it all. Why would nobody listen to me? Why was I not allowed to just be mummy? Why? Why? Why? In my confused state I found the answer; I decided that I wanted to try for another baby before the business really swallowed me up, but Colin had other plans.

CHAPTER 7

Let's Keep Adding Fuel to the Fire!

Colin was dead set against the idea. Our son was his fourth child. He'd had three other sons, one of whom he had no relationship with, and the other two he'd left when they were toddlers. They lived with their mother and spent every weekend with us. My weekends, when I wasn't working in the home office, were spent cooking and providing for Colin's extended family and spending no time with Sam. In fact, if ever I joined them in the lounge for a game of something or to watch a film or TV programme I would be told by Colin "You haven't got time to be watching a film, you've got work to do otherwise you'll lose clients."

However, when I was in the office, if his dinner wasn't ready on time or if he needed some clothes washed or it started to rain whilst washing was on the line and he had to fend for himself for a few minutes I'd be told "You never spend time with the family, you're more concerned about your bloody business than you are with us." I couldn't win. Whatever I did was wrong and not good enough, so why on earth did something deep inside me think another child was the answer?

Colin gave me every reason imaginable as to why we shouldn't have another child, most of which were financial and centred upon the loss to the business of me being away from it to have another child, the amount of extra work I would have to put in to ensure we could afford for me to have another child and the additional cost it would take to have someone look after the child. Any suggestion of me stepping away from the business was met with scorn and disdain. I brushed it off and decided that it would happen if and when it was meant to.

Sometime later I was looking for some paperwork in the home office. I'd turned over every file in and on my desk and proceeded to go through the trays on Colin's desk thinking that perhaps he'd picked up what I was looking for, or that I'd put it down on his desk. I shuffled a few papers and spotted a letter with the address of an unfamiliar doctor. I pulled the letter out of the tray and read it, I couldn't believe what I was reading. This letter was confirmation of an appointment Colin had made to have a vasectomy the following week.

I'm not in the habit of reading other people's personal mail, and my initial reaction to reading this letter was not just of shock and anger but also my own deceit. It didn't cross my mind that the only deception taking place was that instigated by Colin. I confronted him with the letter.

"You've got no right reading my personal mail." He said, knowing that I would find it difficult to argue with that point.

"I didn't open it to read it, it was lying there in your in-tray, underneath some other papers. I was looking for a specific document."

"Well you shouldn't be snooping around my in-tray, it's none of your business."

"Any paperwork relating to my business is my business" I responded indignantly "If you don't want your personal mail to be read, you shouldn't leave it lying around amongst business papers. Actually, I don't care about that, what the hell are you doing booking an appointment for a vasectomy without my knowledge? Why did the doctor book an appointment without discussing it with your wife? Surely he has a duty to ensure that a decision like this has been discussed and agreed with all parties and offer counselling or something if it's not?"

I had so many questions buzzing around my head and so many emotions, I couldn't think straight. I felt sick. I had never felt so deceived in my life. Colin laughed and answered my questions with.

"The doctor asked me if I'd discussed it with my wife and what she thought but I told him it's my body and it's none of her business what I do."

Apparently, that had appeased the doctor who had agreed to book the vasectomy. I didn't believe what I was being told and threatened to call the doctor myself. Colin acquiesced. I wasn't sure why, but I felt I'd got a reprieve. He told me he'd cancel the appointment the following day and then gave me his conditions:

"You have six months to catch, if you're not pregnant by then I'm having the vasectomy."

Once again, I was incredulous. Here was Colin, who claimed to love me, putting a timescale on how long I had to fall pregnant. He knew how difficult it had been for me to carry to term, he'd been with me through the disappointment and upset of the previous 5 miscarriages, how could he do this to me?

I argued that he was being unfair and his demands weren't achievable. I argued that the stress I was under in the business wasn't conducive to falling pregnant within that timescale and more to the point, the stress caused to me by our nightmare neighbours was also having a debilitating effect on my already fragile self-confidence and self-esteem.

And, I ventured, there was one other, major factor that we needed to address. It was impossible for me to get pregnant if he continued to refuse to have intercourse with me.

He had been rejecting me more and more often, citing headaches, depression, my very slight weight gain, the client I'd lost, the extra business I'd taken on, the amount of work he had to do to be a dad to his existing four sons, his age, the fact there was a Y in the day, or the moon was in the wrong phase! Those last two are just my interpretations of his excuses. He didn't *actually* say that, but any excuse he could use to avoid having intercourse he would. I was rapidly feeling fat, ugly and unlovable. Despite the constant rejection I was determined to keep on trying. I told myself that if I gave up trying as well then, we were doomed. But try as I might we remained in a sexless marriage for months to come not helped by the fact that he'd go to bed at 9 p.m and I'd join him sometime between midnight and 2 a.m when I'd finished working. I stopped making the effort to finish my work earlier, knowing from experience that he would find some other excuse not to come near me. In times of desperation he would even say things like he didn't like the way I looked at him earlier in the day or he overheard me talking to a male client on the phone and I was sounding familiar or flirtatious. No matter what I did, he found fault with me.

Resigned to the fact that I was unlikely to have another child I threw myself into my work and business, promising that just as soon as I turned a decent profit, I could take a step back and spend more time with Sam. He was growing fast and I was missing out. This isn't what I'd wanted at all, this isn't how married life with a new baby was meant to be! But neither was it supposed to include a husband who refused to work and insisted on his wife being the sole provider and breadwinner. It was like déjà vu. My only source of relief is that at least this husband didn't beat me when he was upset or angry with me. He did however, tell me during our many arguments that I should be grateful that he didn't beat me, and how I should be grateful that he was with me at all given that no-one else would have me!

His vasectomy was cancelled, but so too were my hopes of having a second child. I realised that weekend, that despite all of his assurances before our wedding and in the early days of our marriage, he had no intention of having any more children but had chosen not to be open and honest with me about it. This was just too much for me to take in and I realised that my second marriage was not much better than my first. However, taking responsibility for my choices I told myself, "You've made your bed, you've got to lie in it," and I set about making the best of things.

I could hear various members of my family's comments in my head, "Young people today give up on marriage too easily," "Marriage is for life and it's not always easy," "You've got to take the rough with the smooth and support each other," "It's not like they write about it in the romance novels,"... and so on and so forth. I decided I needed to grow up, shut up and put up and that somehow a way out of this awful mess I'd created would show itself.

Looking around our beautiful 3-bed semi-detached house in a sought-after area, gazing at my beautiful son, I counted my blessings and felt grateful that whilst my marriage felt a sham, my business was driving me into the ground and our neighbours were harassing me to the point where I was too scared to sit in my own back garden or to tend to the front lawn, I did at least have a roof over my head, a beautiful son, a car to get me from A to B, food in our stomachs, a relatively close family and a large and strong business network and a good reputation within the industry throughout the UK. If I had to take control and turn things around on my own, then so be it. I'd do *whatever it takes.*

Not long after the vasectomy incident, there was an incident with our neighbours which resulted in me goading our neighbour to punch me – I desperately wanted a legitimate reason to call the police and it seemed like a good idea at the time! Our neighbours would get drunk every bank holiday and later in the day and into the evening we would hear him beating his wife, or at least that's what it sounded like through the walls and from her screams. Much as I was terrified of our neighbours, I could not stand back whilst a man beat his wife.

I had bravely ventured into our back garden that afternoon. There was an 8-foot fence and conifer trees between us and them, so although I never knew what they were doing I could hear them and they, if they heard me in the garden, would start shouting insults over the fence. Usually I ignored them but on this particular day I responded. I ignored the insults but threw various random comments their way along the lines of; "It takes a big man to get drunk and beat his wife," "What's it going to be tonight? Black eye? Thick lip?" "Go on, drink a bit more, that will make you punch harder." I knew this was neither big nor clever, but I was at breaking point.

I went back indoors, not exactly pleased with myself, but happy that I had been able to retort and not let their insults get the better of me as they usually did. A few minutes later there was a knock at the front door. I answered and there was our neighbour, drunk, in front of me. He started shouting abuse at me and was swaying. Unfortunately, rather than shut the door, I let rip. All my anger and upset at Colin was hurled his way in the manner of abusive insults and I started goading him as I saw his hand clench into a fist.

"Go on, show me what a big man you are, punch me. Come on, you want to hit a woman, here you are (jutting my chin out) take a swipe at this."

You get the gist. There I was, stood at my front door in a lovely sleepy suburb, shouting at him like a fisher woman. I could hear my mother and grandmother in my head, telling me off for being 'common' but I didn't care. I needed to unleash my pent-up anger and frustration and my neighbour got it.

For all his faults Colin, who had been sitting watching TV in the living room, appeared by my side. He'd heard the raised voices and sensed the escalation of the situation and came to my rescue. As well as having been my kick-boxing instructor he was also six foot, five inches tall so most people were intimidated by his size. Our neighbour, as I goaded him, suffered from small-man syndrome. He was only my height (five feet, four inches) and strutted around with his chest puffed out like a peacock. He also drove a very big car, which I found to be a constant source of amusement as I mentally reminded myself that a big car meant, in colloquial terms, that he had a small, useless penis! On this particularly hot bank holiday, he was stood on our driveway looking the epitome of every other British male in the sun: sunburnt, plastered and fat. The opportunity for me to lay into him was really far too good to miss. I'm not proud of myself for it, but it gave me an enormous sense of satisfaction!

Our neighbour starting lurching towards me and my basic kickboxing training kicked in as I adopted fighting stance with my fists raised. Before I could throw a punch at this idiot Colin had sent a jab his way and knocked him down onto the drive. With our neighbour lying prone on the tarmac, Colin then picked me up under his arm and carried me upstairs, dumped me on the landing and told me to stay out of the way whilst he went down to deal with said neighbour. Unfortunately, (or fortunately), we had a window on our upstairs landing which opened onto our drive, so I opened it up and continued my torrent of verbal abuse as Colin tried to negotiate with our neighbour whilst simultaneously trying to tell me to shut up and butt out in a manner that would show that he was supportive of me!

Our neighbour started threatening legal action for assault and called another neighbour, who had been watching the exchange from his lounge window, over. I got on really well with this neighbour and he and the rest of the street were as fed up with our immediate neighbour as we were; his reputation was bad before we even moved in, so I felt some vindication.

"You saw what happened, he punched me and knocked me down." Said nasty neighbour.

"Did he?" Said nice neighbour.

"You know he did, you were watching."

"All I saw was you trying to punch Deborah-Jane and then you fell backwards and knocked your head on the edge of the driveway. You're drunk, why don't you go home."

With a look of exasperation and much grumbling to himself, nasty neighbour wandered back down our driveway and into his own fortified back garden.

This incident, whilst instigated by me, was the straw that broke the camel's back. As we calmed down I said to Colin. "I can't stay here anymore, we have got to move, I want to be out of here by Christmas." House-hunting was added to my list of ongoing projects, and I spent as much time as I could trawling the internet property sites and looking at the listings in the local newspapers. Every property I selected as a possible new home Colin found fault with; too big, too small, too expensive, not in the right location and so on. He eventually decided that we would be unable to get a mortgage because I hadn't been in business long enough to have the relevant accounts to make the application.

Undeterred, I agreed to wait until we could get the mortgage and move to the place that was right for us, rather than just take anything to get away from our neighbours.

Several weeks later, I arrived home from the office to see Colin looking very pleased with himself. "I've bought a house," he told me.

"What do you mean you've bought a house? I thought we'd agreed to wait until we can afford one. We haven't even looked at any houses."

"Well, I thought I'd save you the worry of house-hunting. I've found the house of our dreams, made an offer which has been accepted and our house is going on the market tomorrow."

I was stunned. Having decided to wait until we could get a mortgage there had been little to no further discussion about moving. I had calmed down after my tirade at our neighbours, and whilst I didn't want to stay living next door to them for any longer than I had to, I wasn't going to move just anywhere and give them the satisfaction of knowing they had driven me out.

I liked our house. I loved that we had spent months and months renovating it before our wedding, we were living in our dream home. I loved the garden and had plans for a vegetable patch and fruit bushes when I had the time. It was even big enough for us to get chickens at some point in the future.

In reality, I just wanted to find some way to manage living next door to such awful neighbours, I'd spoken out in frustration but to leave our home or the area we were in? Was I really going to do that?

CHAPTER 8

New House, New Start

This was all news to me, we hadn't discussed the house of our dreams, or potential locations and I certainly wasn't ready to put the house on the market immediately. I might have said I wanted to move in the heat of the moment, but I wasn't prepared to just pack everything and move on a whim. I didn't want to go from the proverbial frying pan into the fire. Colin however, had decided, in this particular instance, to take what I'd said literally and actually try to do something supportive!

As calmly as possible, I asked Colin to show me the new house online. He called up Google maps and showed me the location of the property. It was at least 20 miles further west than we were living, in the back of beyond, in a village I'd never heard of. It was a good half an hour's drive further away from the office and in completely the opposite direction from most of my business. It was also completely remote from family and friends. I wasn't impressed.

Colin assured me I would love it when I saw it. It had 5 bedrooms and a kitchen I would die for and, he excitedly added, "It has a twenty-foot lounge and twenty-foot dining room so you'll be able to host those dinner parties you keep going on about."

I agreed that in terms of the house size it did sound perfect, but the location was about as far removed from where I wanted to live as anywhere. Besides which, why did we want to be so far away from family and friends? As if that wasn't enough he'd spent our entire time together, some 5 years by now, telling me that the particular area this house was located in was, "the arse end of the world."

I really couldn't understand why this area he supposedly hated was now the location of our dream home. Something didn't add up. Reluctantly, I agreed to go and view our new home. It was a grey drizzly morning when we turned the wrong way off the A48 in South Wales and made our way into the back of beyond.

As we drove up the lane towards the location of the house, Colin pointed it out in the distance. I wasn't happy. I didn't like the area we'd driven through. Despite the weather, it was a region of significant depression and austerity and the houses and businesses we drove past were indicative of that. We turned up another lane and headed uphill towards the house.

There was a terrace of about 8 houses to our right with gardens to the front of them, and a makeshift horse paddock on one house. My first impression was that we were driving past a traveller site.

We continued up the hill past another terrace on the left. I couldn't work out how many houses were in this terrace, some had front doors where I thought the back doors were and others had back doors where I thought the front doors were. There were cars parked randomly all over the place and a medley of children's plastic toys dotted about the lane.

Further up the hill we came to 'our' house. The largest in a terrace of 4 of what I later learned were miner's cottages. There was a detached bungalow at the end of the terrace with a large fence and electric gates. To me it looked imposing, sinister and fortified and I didn't get a good feeling from it.

'Our' house was large, grey and foreboding. It seemed dark and overlooked a field in which there were a number of decaying vehicles. I couldn't tell if they were burnt out or just rusting, but there was nothing about the location or the area that was shouting 'dream home'. It was with some trepidation that I walked through the front door of the house.

I stood in the small hallway and immediately knew I didn't want to see any more. I didn't have a good feeling about this house and just knew I couldn't live there.

I've always had *feelings* about places I've moved to which can be extremely annoying for other people, but if a property doesn't feel right then I can't live there. In my twenties I'd lived in London and my flat mate and I had the opportunity to move from our small 2-bedroom flat to a large former convent, but upon viewing it I had such a bad feeling from the hallway that I refused to live there. Instead we moved to a much smaller property which felt better.

This house was the same. I didn't get a good feeling from it and that was even after putting my preconceptions to one side. I am good at looking at things with an open mind, even if I have massive preconceptions. I love nothing more than my preconceived ideas being smashed to pieces and me being pleasantly surprised.

Unfortunately, this wasn't going to be one of those occasions. As I walked through the house that was used as a family home I didn't get a sense of it being a particularly happy home. A brief conversation with the mother hinted at that, although she didn't go into detail, and Colin wouldn't allow me to be alone with her for too long.

Colin could tell I wasn't happy and insisted on conversing as if we were going to be moving in very soon. This was a tactic he often used on me. If he talked as if something had already happened, I'm sure he thought that would convince me that it had.

As far as he was concerned, my visit was just to dot the 'i's' and cross the 't's'.

We drove away and through tears of anger or frustration, I'm not sure which, maybe even despair, I told Colin that I didn't like the house, didn't get a good feeling from it and couldn't see us living there. He told me that there was nothing I could do about it now as 'our' offer had been accepted and the process had started.

I countered that we weren't obliged to proceed until we'd exchanged contracts, but my protests fell on deaf ears.

Colin spun me a sob story about how the family in our 'dream home' were living apart because mum had been promoted with her work and was living away from home through the week, only coming home at weekends. They were selling the house so that they could all move closer to her work and live together again as a family, it wasn't fair or right of me to stop that.

"Put yourself in her shoes," Colin suggested. "How would you feel if you had to live away from us all week? You wouldn't like it. You can get the house of your dreams and help to keep another family together." In an uncharacteristically selfish response I told him I didn't care about the other family, my priority was my family, no-one else's and I didn't want to live in that "god-awful house in that godforsaken place."

But, Colin had other plans.

He had no intention of withdrawing his offer and could already see himself living in this large property in the back of beyond. He even dared to suggest that it could be run as a bed and breakfast and I could serve breakfast each morning before running the existing business. I wasn't sure whether this was a genuine suggestion or not, I had lost my sense of humour and sense of realism by this point.

Despite all of my objections to the new property, he somehow managed to convince me that we should move in and if I still wasn't happy after six months we could put the property back on the market and move out of the area. I remember sitting on the top stair of our house crying as he pushed the mortgage papers under my nose for my signature.

I knew deep in my gut that this was the very last thing I wanted to be doing and should be doing. No matter what I said, he was now just ignoring my objections, he didn't even bother to cajole me with pithy platitudes any more. We were moving and that was that, and if I didn't sign the papers he'd just forge my signature.

My head was spinning, somehow in the last two years I'd gone from being a happy, excited new bride and mum-to-be to a woman incapable of making her own decisions, scared of her own shadow, practically estranged from her son and with a husband who refused to take her thoughts and opinions into consideration.

All this had happened whilst I was taking responsibility for my family, trying to keep a roof over our head and run a business which, by now, supported six other people.

I felt as if I had no control over what I was doing or who I was, but had no idea how it had happened nor how I could get out of this situation. The only thing I could do was just keep moving forward and hope that somehow this would all sort itself out eventually.

Little did I know that *eventually* is precisely when it would get sorted out, and that *eventually* wasn't going to be a very long time coming!

CHAPTER 9

Pay Peanuts, Get Monkeys

I seemed to be providing for everyone other than myself. It felt that everyone else was happy and well looked after apart for me.

I had six staff, all well paid, and significantly higher paid than if they'd gone elsewhere. I'd insisted that if I wanted the best I could get, I had to pay well. I ensured their salaries were comparable to what I'd been earning before I started the business. They were all on a full time equivalent of £30,000 and my office junior was on £8 per hour.

This was 2006/07 and my team were the people who delivered most of the work. Clients who insisted on me undertaking their work were charged £45 per hour. It was ridiculous, who in their right mind would pay that for secretarial/PA services when they could go to a temp. agency for £12 per hour?

However, my clients did. I knew I was good at what I did, and I ensured that between my team and I, we had experience across the board and complemented each other.

This is what our clients bought, and it's what I paid such good salaries for. I also had a husband who insisted he was doing the best he possibly could by being a 'house husband' and helping me in the business. In reality he was pushing me further away from Sam, not doing anything in the house and unbeknown to me at the time, he was sabotaging my business.

I'd helped Colin to purchase his parent's council property on a 'right to buy' scheme whilst he was unemployed, and I was paying the mortgage for them so that they could still live there.

Colin told me that I was investing in our son's future, and that when his parents moved on or died the property would then be rented out until our son became old enough to either live there, or chose to sell it. I blithely believed him when he told me that his parents were worried about my name being on the title of the property, in case I tried to get them to move out of it, should anything happen to the business. I agreed when it was suggested that the title of the property should just be drafted in his name. After all, my name didn't appear on the mortgage for the property so it didn't make much difference did it? No, I decided, it didn't make much difference, it was still me who would be paying for it, what difference did a piece of paper make?

So, my husband was happy, his parents were happy, my team were happy but meanwhile I was desperately unhappy, and it was beginning to show.

I recall visiting a client. He was a farmer who also had a heavy plant business. He'd employed our services to help him get his paperwork in order and put some processes and procedures in place. He and I had hit it off, and he'd insisted that I should be the person who undertook his administration, particularly because it included assisting with his accounts and payroll. He didn't mind at all paying the higher rate to secure my services.

This particular day, I was sat across from him in his large living room, there were papers and files strewn across his coffee table and he was telling me what his plans were, what the issues were with his business that week and asking for my opinion and advice. I started to make some suggestions when he asked, quite bluntly.

"What's wrong Deborah-Jane?" I was shocked and must have looked quite askance because he continued.

"I know something's wrong, you're not your usual self, what's going on?" Whether it was his genuinely concerned manner, the fact that someone was asking me how I was or my shame at being obviously unfocussed on a client's work I don't know but I burst into tears.

He walked over to me, placed his hands on my shoulders and demanded answers in a gentle but no-nonsense sort of way.

"Is he abusing you?" He asked of Colin.

"No." I replied.

"Are there problems in the business?"

"No."

"Is everything alright with your son or your family?"

"Yes."

"Then what is it?"

"We're moving on Saturday, to this place I've never heard of, to a house I can't stand and I can't do anything about it. I wanted to escape my nightmare neighbours, but I didn't want to live there!"

"Why the hell would anyone choose to live there?" He responded when I told him where we were moving to. "Who in their right mind would move you from where you are now to there?"

I'm sure he thought he was helping but he just proceeded to open the flood gates further, finally stopping the tears when he said, "Well you don't have to move, you could just go to your mother's or to a friend." I think I stopped crying from the shock of what he was suggesting.

"No! I can't." I countered. "The van is booked, Sam has even been offered a place in the local school, which I've not even seen yet, and everything is packed and arranged."

"Well, I have a van and a trailer you could borrow if you wanted to."

I remember laughing at this suggestion, thanking him but declining and then apologising for letting my personal life bubble over into my business.

I made my excuses and promised to return the following week and stay an extra hour or two to make up for the time I'd lost.

I drove back to the office silently berating myself for letting my corporate mask slip so disastrously in front of a client, but I couldn't get the words of his offer out of my head. They would keep spinning around my mind for the next few days.

Could I? Would I? Dare I?

CHAPTER 10

Estranged and Strange

The day of the move arrived and we were up bright and early.

It was a Saturday morning and the removal van was due to arrive around 9 a.m. I'd hardly slept the night before, and woke up with a sense of both impending doom and nervous excitement at around 6 a.m. I made some tea and toast for breakfast then, at around 6.30am, I picked up my mobile phone and called my client.

"Is the offer of a van and trailer still available? Could you come over this morning and help me move?"

My client assured me he would finish his early morning farm chores and be with me at around 9.30 a.m. "But, I don't have the trailer. I hadn't heard from you, so I've loaned it to someone else, but I do have a horse box. As soon as I've coupled it to the van I'll come over."

I gave him the address and directions and hung up.

I took my cup of tea from the kitchen to the hallway and stood at the front door where Colin was busy sorting and shifting boxes. I put my tea down and started to move certain boxes into separate piles. In reality, I was moving those boxes that contained my personal possessions to one side so that I could easily load them into the horsebox. I was also trying to locate everything Sam and I would need for a couple of weeks. I didn't intend to leave Colin, but I needed him to understand just how unhappy I was about this move. My protestations up until this point had fallen on deaf ears so I had to take drastic action.

Between the two of us, we spent the next hour or two moving boxes around the ground floor of our house and keeping our son entertained.

Before long the official moving van arrived and Colin started loading boxes and items of furniture onto it. He started to lift one of the boxes from the pile I'd created when I stopped him.

"Don't put any of my stuff on the van, I'm not coming with you. My van will be arriving shortly. We're going to my mother's. I've told you I don't want to live in the new house, I've told you I don't like it, you've refused to listen, I'm not moving in."

My recollection is that he just shrugged. There was certainly no big argument nor attempt to persuade me to go with him.

I'm certain that my recollection of that moment is correct but maybe time has dulled it.

In my mind I'd built it up to be something much bigger but, when the moment came, he didn't seem to care. He was just intent on getting on with the job of moving.

That was the first time I left Colin.

Sam and I turned up at my parent's home, with me having called them en-route and asking them to make some room in the garage for my boxes because Sam and I were coming to stay for a while.

I continued to run the business and Sam continued to attend nursery on the opposite side of the city, whilst I worked out what to do next.

Things went from bad to worse. Unbeknown to me at the time, the client who had helped me with the horse box had separated from his long-term partner a couple of weeks earlier. You can probably tell where this is going.

Whilst I continued to run the business, take Sam to and from nursery and find us a place to live that was equidistant between all of the key places we needed to be; his dad, my office, his nursery and my parents, people over whom I had no control were conspiring to do as much damage as possible to me, my reputation and my business.

Caught up in my own personal drama I was oblivious.

Within a month of going to stay with my parents I had found Sam and I a lovely little 2-bedroomed garden flat in a beautiful rural village, closer to the area that I actually wanted to live in in the first place. I'd managed to develop some sort of routine and was actually feeling happier than I had in a very long time.

My clients were happy, I was happy, Sam was happy. What more could I ask for?

One Saturday night not long after moving into the flat, I woke up at around 2am. I heard a noise coming from the back garden. I lay in bed assuming it was just foxes or badgers snuffling around but then I heard it again, it was a quiet but insistent knocking at my back door.

Frightened but determined that it shouldn't wake Sam I walked through to the kitchen in the darkness, knowing that if I put the lights on whomever or whatever was outside would see me. I could just about make out the profile of a person stood by my back door, it was a male and he was the cause of the knocking.

I stood for a while not knowing quite what to do, but then I realised that I recognised the shadow and the profile of the person. It was the client who had helped me move. I realised that, during the course of our business over the previous weeks, I had told him where I was moving to. There was only one block of flats in that village and only one of them had a garden, it didn't take Sherlock Holmes to deduce where I was living but at 2 a.m?

I opened the door quietly, invited him into kitchen, told him to stay where he was and be quiet while I went and closed Sam's bedroom door and the internal kitchen door in turn. At this stage I was angry, very angry.

"What the hell do you think you're doing?" I barked in a harsh whisper. "Why the hell are you here? And what on earth gives you the right to knock on my door at this time in the morning?"

My only concern at this time was for Sam, I didn't want him to wake up and wonder who this strange man was in our home.

My client was drunk, he'd been out all evening and as he only lived in the next village had decided to walk to see me and tell me how he felt.

"I love you, I only helped you because I want you, you're free now, you can live with me and we can have babies together."

There are not many times in my life that I've been lost for words, but this was one of them.

I hurriedly thought back to the amount of time we'd spent together. Was my confidence and self-esteem so low that I no longer recognised the signs when someone was attracted to me? And if I didn't recognise them, what on earth had I done to make him think they were reciprocated?

Was I really that naïve?

Over the few months I'd been working with this client I'd come to realise that he really wasn't very nice. He ran his business based on fear, blackmail, manipulation, and a massive desire to get one over on any of his competitors, no matter what the cost. He firmly believed that if he flashed enough cash at anyone or anything he could get what he wanted.

Well I had news for him, it wasn't going to work on me!

However, I now recognised that by jumping to his tune business-wise he was expecting me to do his bidding, and whatever else he wanted as he had helped me out. As far as he was concerned I now owed him something!

When we started working together he would call at 9 p.m or   10 p.m of an evening and occasionally he would insist that I delivered some papers to him or collected some from him, meeting him in a pub car-park or a layby somewhere.

Initially I'd refused to meet him and had Colin's support, but the client obviously wasn't used to people saying "no" to him, and threatened to cancel his contract. He was our largest client by a long shot, and Colin decided I should just do whatever he asked, so when the calls came in for me to drop off files or collect paperwork at all hours of the day or night it was deemed acceptable for me to drop everything and rush to some bizarre meeting point in the South Wales countryside.

I knew this was wrong, I knew that this wasn't how business, proper business was done, and I knew that this wasn't how I wanted to do business, nor the sort of person I wanted to do business with, but again I felt trapped.

On the one hand Colin was insisting I jumped to this man's tune as he was a client and we couldn't risk losing his business; on the other hand, I was appalled that we were allowing one client to call the shots outside of business hours.

Inside I was in turmoil. My gut instinct was firing on red alert but I'd been pushed and pulled in so many directions for so long. I was so far away from how I genuinely liked to work, do business and behave that I really didn't know what was normal anymore, and I'd long given up trusting my instincts.

I was continually asking myself 'Is there even such a thing as normal?'

CHAPTER 11

Someone's Watching
Over Me

I bundled my client into the flat. I wasn't prepared to let him stay, but neither did I want to wake Sam up at that time in the morning. At that point the landline rang. I rushed to answer it, cursing whomever was on the other end for potentially waking Sam.

"Hello?" I whispered angrily.

A woman's voice responded "I know he's there with you. I'm telling your husband you're having an affair. You need to be careful, I know where you both live."

I slammed down the phone in horror and disbelief. As if there wasn't enough drama and upset going on in my life it was now turning into a very bad soap opera.

Without much thought about what I was doing, only focussing on getting this man out of my flat, I quickly went to Sam's bedroom and picked him up. He stirred and I shushed him.

"It's ok sweetheart, we're going on a road-trip adventure, go back to sleep, we're going in the car."

I was grateful that I'd often visited my friends around the UK taking Sam with me. I'd always left on a Friday evening and put him in his pyjamas, wrapped in a blanket, with his favourite cuddly toy and he would sleep for most of the trip. I hoped that, as far as he was concerned, this would just be another one of our adventures.

"Get up." I hissed at my client who by now had made his own way into my lounge and was getting quite comfortable on my sofa. "Don't think you're staying there, you're coming with me, I'm taking you home."

His eyes lit up "And if you think for one minute I find this funny you can think again. Don't talk to me, don't look at me and don't you DARE wake Sam up."

Somehow or other I bundled the client and Sam into the car, strapping Sam into his car seat and making soothing noises to send him back to sleep. Within an instant he was gently snoring and chuntering in the way that toddlers do.

My client was also snoring – in the front seat, not doing himself any favours! I drove the six miles to his farm and pushed and pulled him out of the passenger seat as we got to the gate. By this time he had managed to sober up a little and I think the reality of what he had done, where he was and what was happening, was slowly beginning to dawn on him. He started to talk to me, but I shut him up.

"Just go home, we'll discuss this tomorrow or Monday." I drove off, shaking with fear, anger and surprise. I was angry with him for trying to take advantage of me, angry with myself for not seeing any of the warning signs and surprised by how I'd handled him. One thing was certain, my mothering

instinct was very much front and centre, and woe betide anyone who might put me and Sam in danger.

But those feelings soon turned to worry and anxiety. What if my client cancelled his contract? What if my client didn't cancel his contract but tried to control me? What if that woman on the end of the phone really did speak to Colin? What if? What if? What if?

I started to berate myself; "You should have let him stay, he was drunk, it's not as if he was capable of anything. Why did you have to be so rude to him? What will your husband say? How are you going to face the client again? How could you possibly have led him on to think you might welcome his advances? Why did you put yourself and your son in this position? Stupid, stupid woman, who the bloody hell do you think you are? You should know you're not capable of being on your own, you're a risk to yourself and to your son."

It went on, by the time I'd finished with all my self-talk, it was my fault that the client was on my doorstep, and it was my fault that I'd been put in that position. I really couldn't see that any blame could be apportioned to my client. When eventually we did talk the following week it was me apologising to him for being so rude to him.

But that was the least of my problems.

The following weekend I walked back into the flat after hanging some washing on the line to hear Sam talking to someone.

I had left him watching CBeebies whilst I was in the garden putting the washing out and initially assumed he was talking to the TV. As I walked into the living room I saw that he was on the phone. I took the phone out of his hand and said, "Hello." The female voice on the other end chilled me.

"What a lovely little boy you have, so friendly, so polite, it would be awful if something happened to him."

"Who is this?" I asked but the caller had put the phone down.

I dialled 1471 but the number was withheld. Over the course of the next 10 days I received numerous other calls, some silent, others commenting on what a busy day I'd had, darting here, there and everywhere in my little red Tigra.

My car was noticeable, apart from being a red Tigra I'd also had it sign-written with the company logo and contact details. This person seemed to know exactly where I had been and at what times. It was unnerving to say the least.

Then I received a call from an unrecognised number on my mobile. I always answered those calls because they might be business enquiries.

The voice on the other end started to accurately describe my parents' home and garden, what my parents looked like and the clothes Sam was wearing, they also described my niece. I recognised the voice to be the same as the woman who had been calling my house. Within minutes, I had called my office, cancelled the rest of my appointments and was making my way to my parents' home to check that everyone was all right.

En-route I also had an irate call from my estranged husband.

"I don't know what the hell is going on with you and your client and I don't care, but when his ex-wife turns up on my doorstep and lets herself into my garden whilst I'm outside I want to know. If you're putting our son at risk I need to know about it."

At that point I realised I knew exactly who was behind all the phone calls. My client's ex-partner had underestimated the relationship Colin and I had and had assumed that it was as acrimonious as hers with my client. It wasn't. We were determined to do the right thing for our son and we were determined to keep things as amicable as possible. Neither of us at this stage had ruled out a reconciliation and we were very much still friends. I asked him to meet me at my flat in an hour or so when I had collected our son and returned home.

That was an interesting conversation!

I told Colin about the telephone calls and about the visit from my client. I was totally open and honest with him about the relationship I had with the client. Yes, we were friends and yes, I was helping him out to the extent of even doing some shopping for him at Tesco one day and helping him to clean his farmhouse and get himself sorted out, as he hadn't really looked after himself since his partner left him.

No, I wasn't having an affair and all the time I was disappearing at odd hours to deliver some paperwork, which Colin could have done but refused. I was scared that if I didn't do as I was asked (or told) I would lose my largest client, which meant that not only could I have not paid the mortgage on our marital home, I would now be unable to contribute towards the mortgage on the new house that I was yet to live in, nor pay the rent on the flat I was living in. Colin urged me to go the police.

I contacted them and they arrived to take a statement from me which, they assured me, they would follow up and report back to me. I'm convinced now that Colin only suggested I went to the police to check whether I was telling the truth or not, knowing that I wouldn't lie to the police.

Sometime later I received a call from my client. To say he was irate was an understatement.

"Why didn't you ask me to sort it out?" He ranted, "You didn't need to go to the police, I would have had a word with her."

I reminded him that I had already asked him to have a word and things had got worse.

He was furious that I had gone to the police and the thought crossed my mind that maybe it was him feeding her information about me. He had, after all, gained my confidence by helping me to move out, he and I had become each other's confidantes whilst working together, he was getting to know an awful lot about me and my family and the situation with Colin. As quickly as the thought appeared in my mind, I shut it down. There's no way he would do that I told myself. Why would anyone do something like that?

It transpired that the police had visited his ex-partner, who was known to them for previous similar behaviour and she had spent an evening in police custody being questioned. They visited me the following day and asked me to press charges. I spoke to Colin about it and we decided that I wouldn't press charges as I was worried about repercussions from my client in terms of my business. I even told my client that I had chosen not to press charges because I didn't want it to damage our business relationship. With hindsight, sharing that snippet of information was a really bad idea.

In that instant, in those few words, I had given the client the opportunity to control me, and he used it as much as he possibly could.

The incident did have its uses however as it enabled Colin and I to talk about our future. He came and ate dinner with me and our son and stayed the night. A few nights later, I visited and stayed at his (our) house. Whilst I still didn't like the house, it did, on this particularly sunny day, seem a lot more welcoming than it had on the day I viewed it. It wasn't long before we both decided to reconcile and I served notice on my flat and moved into the house that I'd vowed I wasn't going to live in.

This was October 2008, some three months after we had moved from our beautiful home in order to escape our nightmare neighbours.

CHAPTER 12

Starting Over

After I moved in with Colin again things seemed to improve.

I was able to create a home office, and although Colin was still a house-husband I had a good team in place and I was able to leave them to get on with their work whilst I met potential clients, carried on networking and caught up on business at home.

I spent perhaps an hour a day in the actual office and most of the rest of my time was either spent on the road or in the home office.

Although I felt increasingly isolated at home, I just couldn't face the commute to the office which would take me through both the area we lived in and the area that I really wanted to live in. It just served to upset me, and with a team in place that I could depend upon I became more and more distant from my business premises and spent more and more time working from home.

In the November I had an accident which meant I was housebound until Christmas. I slipped off the bottom stair as

I was going downstairs. I thought I had twisted my ankle but couldn't move and had to wait until Colin arrived home from the swimming pool with our son to help me get into a chair.

A quick trip to the local A&E revealed that I had torn the ligaments in my left ankle. I was in plaster up to the knee and given crutches to help me get about. There was no way I could drive anywhere, so I had to run my business and undertake as much networking as possible from home.

These were the days before Twitter or Facebook became prevalent, so I had to utilise email and Skype as much as I could and I spent a lot of time on the telephone.

Colin helped in as much as he looked after our son so that I could carry on running the business. He would chip in with suggestions, and shortly before my accident I had asked him to come back into the business and assist me. Things were tough financially, and I needed to get out and about and drum up more business whilst implementing a new marketing campaign.

The weekend that we had moved from our marital home and gone our separate ways also coincided with another office move.

Colin had, once again, found a larger office which we could grow into. Again, the cost was significantly more than we could afford but it was in a much more central location. In his defence, we had been given notice on our first office as the building it was in was part of a compulsory purchase order which had been granted on the land it was built on. We had very little choice, although we didn't need to move to quite such a large office.

However, I had allowed myself to be talked around and to view it as future-planning. Once again Colin convinced me that if we continued to grow at the rate we had grown so far, we would soon need the space.

So, now that I was incapacitated, I was more dependent upon Colin than ever. He was visiting the office daily after dropping our son off at pre-school.

I had sat down with him and run through the marketing strategy and we had a weekly plan of what needed to happen. Much of it was online marketing, a relatively new strategy and marketing method at the time, but I wanted to back it up with some direct marketing and needed my team to prepare mailshots and make follow up calls.

The plan was to send out 50 letters per week to a carefully selected target market and then follow them up the following week with a phone call so that in any given week we were making 100 contacts. I had purposefully set it up in this way, so that each of my team could make a couple of calls each. I was available to have Skype consultations with anyone who was interested in progressing further.

I didn't want to do a mass mailing, as I would be unable to manage any growth and would lose momentum if I was unable to physically visit potential clients when they requested. I was secretly grateful that Christmas was around the corner as I knew that most people would book meetings for after Christmas. By then, I would be driving again and could take up the helm.

The time and money I had invested in a freelance Marketing Director was really paying off. She totally understood our business, understood how I liked to work and related to our target market. Between us both we were able to come up with some creative ideas to generate engagement from the mailings and even found some target markets I'd never even considered.

Working with someone who was an expert in their field combined with my sometimes 'wacky' creativity was doing me the world of good and I knew it would help to grow the business.

What I didn't know was that Colin didn't buy into the new marketing strategy and had ideas of his own that weren't shared with me.

CHAPTER 13

A Christmas and New Year, Never to Forget

It seemed that Christmas was upon us in no time at all.

I had managed to get through November and December. My clients had all received the work they were expecting by their deadlines, some marketing had been undertaken, invoices were issued and debts were being chased. Whilst not quite in the position I would have liked to have been in, I knew it could have been worse and I was quietly pleased that we had managed to get this far without any major disaster. I knew that the 2-week break over Christmas would be the time I needed to fully relax and recover properly. I contacted the office and wished my team Season's Greetings and told them to have a good break and relax. I also confirmed with them that they wanted to receive their salaries on New Year's Eve. I always paid them on the last day of the month but in December I gave them the choice whether they had it prior to Christmas or on the last day as usual. All of them asked for payment on the last day so that the next month wasn't a long one.

I spent the Christmas period planning a large family lunch, which turned out to be the last my grandmother would attend, and I generally looked forward to being the hostess.

We had a fabulous Christmas., My in-laws stayed over on Christmas Eve, and as usual Colin set up the video camera so that he could film our son opening his presents on Christmas morning. As usual, he sat in front of the camera with our son on his lap and me just out of shot. I had become used to this on Christmas mornings, telling myself it was all about our son. Colin would often tell me our son was more relaxed and happy sitting on his lap because he was around him all day. It would send daggers into my heart, but I learned to shrug it off.

Over time I became deaf to the comments about me never being around and him being the better parent. I knew they weren't true, but there was no point arguing over it. It always came back around to the same argument, that I had the greater earning potential and he was far more comfortable around children than I was. I was left to be the hostess and make bacon sandwiches for him and the in-laws and a smoked salmon bagel for me, washed down with a glass of champagne. I always treated myself to a bottle of champagne for Christmas Day. I'd have a glass with my smoked salmon bagel for breakfast and then finish the rest of the bottle from lunchtime onwards.

With presents opened I became a recluse in the kitchen, washing dishes and getting lunch going. As well as my in-laws we were expecting my parents, my grandmother, my sister and my niece. There would be 10 of us for lunch, I was really looking forward to it. I love to entertain people and there was no reason why I shouldn't enjoy the rest of the day, opening presents was just a small part of it.

In his usual fashion I had absolutely no say in what 'we' had bought our son for Christmas, so I had no idea what he would be unwrapping. As usual the gifts were not age appropriate, he always bought him gifts that were a year or two too old for him, using our son's 'outstanding intelligence' as his reason. After all, we wanted to keep him engaged and challenged so that he could go out and earn millions when he was older.

He hadn't been there when his other three sons were growing up and was adamant that our son wouldn't miss out on his superior parenting skills, believing that their mothers were lazy and not spending enough time with his sons to give them a proper education. I couldn't argue against that, I didn't know the other mums well enough and I certainly wasn't around as I was running the business.

Christmas Day came and went much like any other day and Boxing Day was spent between my parents' home and my in-laws who put on cold spreads for the wider family and friends. I really love spending time with family and friends and to be able to do so over the Christmas period, when I had some proper down-time, was a treat for me. I was starting to feel relaxed and energised ready to start again in early January 2009.

The next few days were a whirl of entertaining visitors and visiting other friends and family before we started to plan for New Year's Eve.

I'd never been a fan of New Year's Eve, it had too many negative connotations for me that were hungover from my first, physically abusive marriage. I was always quite happy to treat it as just another day, watch Jools Holland's Annual Hootenany on the TV, drink a glass of wine or champagne at midnight and go to bed, if I even managed to stay awake until then. We were planning pretty much the same for this New Year, although I was going to prepare a nice dinner for just the two of us that evening.

New Year's Eve dawned quite grey and drizzly and I set about preparing food for my small family. We ate breakfast and generally pottered around with me taking the Christmas tree and decorations down. I always like to start the New Year with a clean house and the detritus of the previous year either packed away or thrown away. It was mid-morning, around 11am before I remembered I needed to pay my team. I went into the office and sat at the computer, logging into the business banking and pulling out the relevant cards, books and payroll information I needed.

Sipping a coffee, I waited whilst the bank accounts loaded. We had three bank accounts in total; one for our main business, one for a sister company which offered similar services to Tradespeople and a tax account to set aside our tax ready for the end of the financial year.

The tax account said exactly what I was expecting it to say, the sister company account didn't have much in it, it rarely did. This was the company that had been set up for Colin to manage as he was more comfortable talking to tradespeople than the executives who I targeted. The main business account didn't show what I was expecting.

Deciding that I had made a mistake, I logged out and straight back in again but the accounts still read the same. There wasn't enough money in the accounts to enable me to pay my salaries. I reached for the invoices folder to manually tot up what I had invoiced earlier in the month.

Yes, I had invoiced the correct amount and yes, they were all set up on Standing Order. Why wasn't the money there? I called the bank and had an interminable wait to speak to a human being. It transpired that a small number of standing orders had been cancelled in the last week and I hadn't yet received the letters notifying me of that as the Christmas post was unreliable. I was given the list of cancellations and checked them against the invoices I had issued, they added up. I was about £1,000 short to enable me to pay my salaries.

Feeling sick and starting to see stars in front of my eyes I called the bank again. No, they couldn't extend my overdraft or give me a loan without me having a meeting with my account manager. No, he was on holiday and I wouldn't be able to see him for another week. Yes, they were sorry about the situation but there was nothing they could do to help. With panic setting in, it dawned on me that my business was insolvent.

I Googled 'insolvency' and the definitions I found confirmed that I was correct. My business was insolvent. I knew I needed some expert advice and I needed it fast. I needed to pay some salaries today. My team all had various New Year's Eve events to attend and they were looking forward to having some money to spend.

Checking my personal bank account and credit card, I knew that I didn't have the funds there but I was praying that somehow I'd made a mistake and not spent as much as I thought I had on Christmas. If only I could find some spare money somewhere. There was about £200 available on my credit card, but it wasn't enough. I wondered if Colin might have some spare money languishing in one of his accounts but decided against asking him. He never had any spare money if I asked him for some help with the household expenses, although he always had plenty if either of his teenage sons needed some.

Going back to Google I typed in 'insolvency advisors'. I wasn't sure if I'd be able to speak to anyone on New Year's Eve, but I needed to try. The first few numbers listed had out of hours messages on their answerphones, finally, by about the fifth or sixth attempt, I got an answer from a real human being.

I explained the situation and asked for advice, I had no idea what to do next. The faceless voice gave me some very clear instructions and after taking what little money I could part with as payment for his 'manage your own insolvency and administration' instruction manual he advised me that if I continued to trade I was breaking the law.

I was left with no choice but to "call your staff and make them redundant with immediate effect and no pay. Then call your debtors and try to enter in a voluntary agreement with them. "But," and he stressed this point, "You can only enter into a voluntary agreement if every single one of them agrees to it, you cannot pay any one of them a single penny until you have reached an agreement that they are ALL happy with. If they don't all agree you will have to put your business through administration and probably declare yourself bankrupt. As you have no money to pay someone to do it for you, you will have to do it yourself."

I didn't think it was possible for your life to pass before your eyes if you weren't dying, but I'm sure that my life passed before my eyes at that moment. I thought about the fun Christmas we'd had, my family's happy, smiling faces, Sam full of excitement at having the whole family over for a 'party'. I thought of the lovely time we'd spent visiting friends and family and having them visit us. It didn't seem possible that events had taken such a drastic turn within 24 hours. Surely, I was having a bad dream? But I knew that I wasn't.

I called Colin, I think the tone of fear and panic in my voice had him flying up the stairs into the office within seconds. I told him what the situation was and waited. He stood rooted to the spot, back against the wall, just inside the door, his hands were hanging limply by his side as I asked him,

"Please just give me a hug and tell me it will be ok, that we'll get through this." I'll never forget the look on his face nor the look in his eyes as he said,

"I can't, I don't know that we will." And then he really tore into me.

"I told you this would happen, what made you think you could run a business? You don't have what it takes, you're not fit to be a businesswoman. You've been out there pretending all this time whilst it's been me who's run your business. You're an embarrassment and a disappointment. Nobody likes you, everybody knows it's me who's made this business work, they're all laughing at you. They'll find this hysterical when they find out the mess you've made of it."

That was the moment that I knew my second marriage was over!

"I'm not expecting you to fix it." I said. "I just need a hug from you right now and then I can sort it out."

"No, you need to get on the phone to the girls," he said handing me the phone. I dialled the number of my office junior.

"Hi." She answered brightly, recognising my number on her mobile. "I'm so excited, we're getting ready to go out tonight...blah, blah, blah."

I have no idea what else she said because I broke down. I couldn't talk, my mouth and tongue were moving but no words were coming out. In the end Colin took the phone from me and told her,

"I'm sorry, she's fucked up, the business is insolvent and has to close. She's ringing to tell you you're redundant with immediate effect and no pay. Sorry, Happy New Year."

Understandably she was shocked, she had a few more words of conversation with Colin and then they hung up.

The same scenario was repeated another five times, each time it felt like the knife was twisted just a little bit further. I don't think I could have felt more pain if Colin had actually stabbed me with a bread knife. I thought I'd felt lonely in my marriage before, now I felt completely abandoned. I was on my own, alone, in this god-awful house and I had only myself to depend upon. Colin walked out of the room and said. "I'm taking Sam out, so you can sort out this mess."

I was all alone and needed to work out what I was going to do.

The following week was a whirl of calling debtors and creditors. I contacted each of the three clients who had failed to pay us and asked them why.

Without exception they responded with, "I wanted to keep the money in our account over Christmas, you can have it next week." Without exception I advised them that "next week is too late, the company is now in administration, the team have been made redundant with immediate effect and no pay. You will have to find someone else to undertake your business administration and secretarial services and you can no longer access your online calendar."

I'm not sure what I expected them to say or do but I recall feeling shocked by how apathetic they were to the predicament.

The general response I got was a metaphorical shrug of the shoulders and an, 'Oh well, that's just business', I couldn't believe it. I'd built up a relationship with these clients over the time we'd worked with them and yes, I hadn't been around much in the months leading up to Christmas, but I had been in telephone and email contact with them.

Those few months of not having face-to-face contact had led them to devalue our relationship and feel as if I had depersonalised the service they were receiving. Despite it being nobody's fault, after all these things happen, they had treated me in the way they treated any other 'faceless' business. They needed the money to assist their cash-flow over Christmas and as they hadn't physically seen me for a while they had decided I didn't value them.

The remaining clients all cancelled their standing orders upon my instruction but agreed to continue working with me if the business was to carry on. I told them that I would have to wait for the outcome of the conversations with my debtors before being able to work with them. I must have had a sixth sense that things weren't going to go quite as I hoped.

For the most part, my conversations with our debtors weren't as bad as they could have been. My intention was to enter into voluntary arrangements with them and pay back as much as possible by working my way out of the hole we were in. Most clients were still happy to work directly with me on a reduced service.

All of the debtors, bar one, agreed a voluntary arrangement. The majority of the debtors were sympathetic to our plight and were grateful that I'd called them and been open and honest with them. It meant that they would get more, if not all, of what they were owed rather than if I had just declared bankruptcy.

Unfortunately, because just one debtor didn't agree I had no choice but to pursue administration of the business. The law at the time stated that if you were unable to pay back all of your debtors at the same time then you had to go into administration. I asked the bank for help knowing deep down that they wouldn't be at all supportive. The bank had never truly understood my business, insisting it was a lifestyle business even when I had six employees and was smashing all turnover and sales goals.

All the bank saw was a business they could sell to and boy did they try to sell! Numerous products we didn't need were offered and would have driven us into debt much quicker than any other impact on the business. In truth, I believed what they were doing was unethical and questioned them about it on a number of occasions. As it turned out, it was the bankers who were globally blamed for the recession that we were on the brink of at that time. I hold no grudge, the people I was dealing with were just doing their job, but I will never bank with that particular bank again for the rest of my life. I had asked for an emergency overdraft increase of just £500 to enable me to pay my staff and keep my business going. Now, just 2 weeks after them declining that small amount, I was in the position of having to close the business because of one debtor. The total sum owed to him was around £1,500. The more I tried to negotiate, the more aggressive the client became. I was immediately referred by him to a debt collection agency. At one stage I was receiving ten or more telephone calls per day, pursuing me for money I didn't have. Each time I remained polite and firm, advising them that if their client had accepted my offer of a voluntary arrangement they wouldn't be in this position and I wouldn't be outright refusing to pay a single penny. I was incensed, I was being bullied and harassed by these people because I'd been upfront and honest and wanted to do the right thing. It wasn't the first time I was 'low hanging fruit' and unfortunately it wasn't the last either. I was rapidly coming to the conclusion that perhaps honesty wasn't the best policy after all.

I would rue my honesty plenty of more times in later years.

CHAPTER 14

A Glimmer of Hope

In the midst of all the upset and the negotiations taking place in those first few weeks of 2009, I kept in contact with the clients who had paid me and were so far standing by me. I kept them appraised of the situation and completed as much work as I could for them. I also set about trying to find them new virtual PAs or administrative support.

Word was spreading fast in the business networks I belonged to, it didn't take long before I was receiving email and telephone requests to sell my client list and contacts. I was adamant I wasn't going to sell my contacts, I might be in dire straits but that didn't excuse me for selling out on my morals and ethics. I knew I had a good reputation and I wanted to keep it that way. To this day, I've never sold a single contact list.

Most are now obsolete this far after the event, but I still have a good network and retain contact with those whom I trust and to whom I pass possible leads. Networking and connecting people is something I've done for years, almost without realising it. I see links between what people do, meet people whom I believe would and could work well together and put them in touch. If they end up working together great, if not, it's cost them an hour of their time and a cup of coffee. No-one has ever asked me to stop sending referrals their way and it's not something I felt I would stop just because I no longer had a business.

My clients on the other hand were a different kettle of fish. All so different and all worked with different members of my team as suited their personalities and business needs. I prided myself on connecting them with the right person for the job as well as the right person for them.

Years of being a corporate PA had taught me that even the best PA in the world wouldn't shine if she and her boss didn't get on well. I ended up interviewing by telephone the majority of the VAs who had contacted me, and gradually I was able to pass recommendations to my clients. I'm happy that most of my clients chose to work with the person who had been my first choice for them. To this day, I'm still in touch with many of my former clients whose businesses have continued to grow from strength to strength.

One of my clients however had a different proposition; how would I like to join him on a self-employed basis and become his Business Development Director? We met and discussed the requirements of the job, the terms of the contract and my fees. These were agreeable to both parties and it didn't take long for me to accept his offer. By now it was mid-February and I needed to get an income. Colin of course, wasn't working and was looking to me to sort out the mess that I'd created. He had by now washed his hands of anything to do with the business. I will never forget his response to me telling him about the job offer from my client.

We were busy preparing for Colin's 40th birthday. We didn't have the money to enable us to splash out on a large party, but we were in a large house and I could cook. I had just about £100 to my name and suggested we invite 16 friends over for dinner (we could seat 20 people around our table), and I would cook a birthday meal. I'd received the job offer and had the meetings with my client through the week and he'd emailed me confirmation of his offer and the terms that morning. It was a Saturday. All of the friends were contacts we'd made through business and they were people that Colin knew.

However, on the Saturday morning he decided he was depressed and couldn't get out of bed, he wasn't sure if he was strong enough to attend his party. I was annoyed but kept quiet.

I had spent the whole day on the Friday shopping for and preparing the food we would eat; a starter of Parma ham and fig salad, followed by slow roasted lamb shanks, mashed potato and seasonal veg and finishing with a shop prepared dessert of chocolate gateaux. I'd also prepared stuffed aubergines for the vegetarian diners and replaced the Parma ham in their starter with honeydew melon. I'd bought a couple of bottles of wine, not much as Colin didn't drink and most people would be driving, but enough for everyone to have at least one glass. It was quite a simple meal but preparing it for 20 people was no mean feat. I was determined that we would make his milestone birthday one to remember and try to forget, for a few hours, the events of recent weeks.

On the Saturday morning, I still had a few errands to run and had asked Colin if he would run the hoover over and clean the bathroom whilst I was out. As soon as I returned from my errands, I needed to start cooking and set the table. Colin, deciding he wasn't well enough to get up, also said that he wouldn't be able to help with the housework. I asked him if he wanted me to cancel the guests, but he refused as we had so much food in the house and they would have planned to attend. It was still early enough in the day (before 10am) for me to call everyone to cancel and I told him that we could sort out the food. We could eat some of it ourselves over the next day or two and the rest could go into the freezer. I was more than happy to prepare the vegetables and freeze them so nothing would go to waste.

Again, he refused for me to cancel the guests, so I carried on. Sam came with me on our errands for Daddy's birthday and then he helped me with the housework and preparation. I made a game of it as much as I could, he was only 3 at the time and inordinately excited at the prospect of a proper grown up birthday party.

By late afternoon, I had things under control and at 5.30pm I asked Colin to get up and keep an eye on things whilst I went upstairs to change, knowing that I wouldn't get much chance in the next hour as I had so much going on in the kitchen. He got up and got dressed but rather than keeping an eye on things as I'd asked, he informed me he was going out. When I asked him where he was going he informed me he was going to collect his two teenage sons as he wanted them there at his birthday and we had plenty of food, so 2 more people wasn't going to make much difference. He took Sam with him to collect his half-brothers.

At 7pm, with guests starting to arrive, Colin was nowhere to be seen. I told guests that he was obviously stuck in traffic having gone to pick up his other two boys. Thankfully, our guests were all good friends and those that arrived first helped me to answer the door and pour drinks, I joined them in what was my first glass of wine of the evening. At around 7.15pm, as I was starting to think the food would be spoiled Colin, Sam and his half-brothers arrived. I asked Colin where he had been as I was getting worried about him and his flat response was, "I wanted to spend my birthday with my boys, we only came back because of all the food." I tried to let his comment go over my head, but inwardly I was seething. I'd bent over backwards to give him a birthday celebration, I'd agreed everything with him, he'd selected who he wanted to invite and I hadn't said a word about him staying in bed all day.

He didn't even know that I'd had a firm offer of work from my client. I busied myself getting everyone to sit down and I brought the food out. The chatter and camaraderie around the table was good but Colin wasn't interacting with anyone other than his three boys. It was becoming extremely noticeable and embarrassing and I'm sure many of the guests only stayed as long as they did out of politeness for the amount of time and effort that had gone into the meal. At around 8.45pm, almost as soon as he'd finished eating dessert but not before everyone else had finished, Colin stood up and said he was going as he had to take the boys home. Everyone was surprised but tactfully carried on with their conversations. I suggested that the boys could stay the night if he just called their mum, they had brought their night clothes with them, so it had always been a possibility. I also told him that he hadn't heard my good news. He asked me what it was.

"I've had a written offer of work from my client (giving the name), he wants me to start on Monday and is paying me £2,000 per month. Everything's going to be OK." A number of the friends closest to us had heard what I'd said and congratulated me. There were various platitudes and murmurs of congratulations and relief that hopefully we could start to look to the future.

Colin looked at me as if he was looking at someone he despised and commented, for all to hear, "You've obviously been sleeping with him, why else would he offer you a job like that on that sort of salary? No-one else wants to work with you, that can be the only reason."

Needless to say, it caused the utmost embarrassment and discomfort to all present. My jaw hit the floor. I couldn't believe Colin would think so little of me. I was presenting him with a solution to our problems and all he could say was he thought I was sleeping with the client.

For a split second my world stopped once more, but quickly I came back to my senses and realised we were now playing this out in front of friends and my step-sons.

I responded with, "I can't believe you think that of me, I thought you'd be pleased. You'd better take the boys home, I'll tell you more about the job when you get back." With that he left with his two eldest sons. I was grateful Sam was in bed and hadn't witnessed how little his father thought of me. As Colin drove off, the majority of our friends made their excuses and left.

There were cursory offers to assist with tidying up, which I declined wanting to take my frustration out on the various chores that follow a dinner party. The last couple to leave were a business contact and his wife. He had been one of the first people I'd met when I'd started my business and we had become good friends. They had arrived earlier with a bottle of Chateauneuf du Pape and I asked them if they'd like to join me in a glass. Colin didn't drink and it would be nice to share such a lovely bottle of wine with friends.

I was glad that they agreed to stay and between the three of us we drank the bottle, tidied up and chatted generally. My friend and his wife offered much support if I needed it and told me to call them if I needed to talk and then they left. No sooner had they gone, than Colin arrived back with a face like thunder. I asked him what the matter was, and he told me he was "disappointed." I asked what about and he responded, "You. You're pissed."

"I had one glass of wine whilst I was preparing dinner, one with dinner and have just shared a bottle of wine with our friends, I'm hardly pissed," was my indignant response.

He looked at me again as if he despised me and said, "I'm going to bed I don't want to look at you."

I asked. "What on earth has got into you? I don't understand why you're being like this." To which he responded as he pushed past me.

"You can sleep in the spare room, I don't want you near me."

"I see," I said. "This is about the job offer isn't it? Why on earth do you think I would sleep with a client just to get a job?"

"Because you're desperate. Why else would he offer you such a good job?" was Colin's response.

This was just another body blow and I decided that no matter what I said he wouldn't believe me. I knew I hadn't slept with the client. I had always made it a rule that I didn't mix business with pleasure. It was a rule I lived by from my very first day in my very first job. I certainly wasn't going to get myself a reputation for getting business because I slept with clients. I knew that I'd got the jobs I got and the client list I'd built because I was good at my job.

No amount of bickering, pleading or debating with Colin was going to change his mind and I'd just run out of energy to argue any more. I left him to go up to bed and finished clearing and tidying away. I made a cup of tea then took that and a glass of water up to the spare bedroom. I eventually fell asleep and awoke the next morning when Colin brought me a cup of tea and Sam leapt on me. I thanked Colin for my tea and asked him what we were going to do today. He responded with "I don't know, I'm not talking to you." I turned my attention to Sam who was asking a flurry of questions.

"Why are you sleeping in the guest bedroom mummy?" "Will you come and play?" "Can we go to the park?" He was still high on the excitement of Daddy's birthday party.

I put my arms around him and suggested he went and got a book and I'd read him a story, then he could help me put all the dishes away out of the dishwasher and we would make some breakfast. I was in distraction mode. I knew what Colin was like when he decided not to talk to someone, I'd seen him do it often enough to various family members. He hadn't spoken to one of his sisters for over 2 years, moving out of the room if she entered the same room he was in when at family events. I had often asked him how he found the energy to be so angry, but he always had some sort of excuse about how it was the other person's fault for saying or doing something 'disrespectful' about him or to him.

We had had plenty of arguments about him chastising our son and saying to him, "that's naughty, go away, I'm not talking to you." Our son would end up distraught and eventually, within around 48 hours Colin would start talking to him again. I argued that it wasn't showing our son the correct way to handle disagreements or misbehaviour but no matter how much I tried to reason with him Colin insisted he was right and I was wrong, reminding me time and time again, "What do you know? You've never had children before."

I was constantly reminded that my mothering skills were far from adequate and I was genuinely grateful that I'd married such an expert despite feeling deep down that I actually did know what I was doing. It was imperative to me that Sam didn't see the disharmony between his dad and I. There had been enough negative emotion in the air over recent months and I was determined that this job offer would mark a new positive start for us. I ignored everything my gut instinct was screaming at me. I told myself that everything would be alright eventually, that Colin was just feeling overwhelmed and worried.

I prayed to whoever was listening that things would work out soon.

CHAPTER 15

Fresh Start

One week after the dinner party I was still sleeping in the guest bedroom and Colin was still not talking to me. He would walk out of any room he was in if I entered it and we had spent a week doing this ridiculous dance. I was grateful that over the years I had developed skin like a rhino. It was something I'd always joked about in my various PA roles. I was first in the line of fire for my boss's bad mood or the anger of a client or co-worker directed at whichever company or boss I happened to be working for. I'd learned not to take it personally, but this was tiring. It was hard after a week of Colin ignoring me not to take it personally. I'd had enough.

I started to think about alternatives. I'd been working in my new job for a week and it all seemed to be going well. Life looked as if it was improving. I decided that if Colin wasn't going to change then I needed to. I was going to try to talk to him this evening (it was a Friday) and if he still refused to talk to me then I would have no choice but to leave. It would be obvious whether or not he wanted to remain married to me or to try to improve things. I knew that I was pushing for a solution and he possibly wasn't ready to have that conversation, but I couldn't spend any more time living in a house I'd never wanted to live in, in an area I really didn't like, knowing no-one and with a husband who refused to talk to me. The only reason for me being there was Sam and he was becoming more and more withdrawn. He had often asked me, "Why are you sad mummy? Why are you crying mummy?" and where once these questions had started to ebb away, they were now becoming daily, almost hourly questions. These shouldn't be the words that a 3-year old said most often. I knew that for the benefit of Sam I had to take action of some sort. It wasn't healthy for him to have two parents who didn't talk, what sort of example would that give him of how to conduct a relationship?

I had two plans;

Plan A - if Colin wanted to work on our marriage I would insist that he came back to the couples counselling we had started but he'd walked away from saying, "There's nothing she can tell me that I don't already know" and "It's obvious she's biased towards you, you knew her and booked the sessions."

or

Plan B - I would leave. I would go and stay with my parents initially. They didn't really have room, but I could stay there for a short while as I had done before and find a flat near to them whilst organising pre-schooling for Sam. When the schooling was organised I would go back and get Sam, but for the time being I didn't want to disrupt his routine. He was in the local village pre-school and thoroughly enjoying it. He had been disrupted enough in the past year. I didn't want to uproot him again until I knew I was settled and he was taken care of. I anticipated everything being organised within a week to 10 days.

That evening, when I arrived home from my new job, whilst preparing dinner, I rehearsed what I was going to say. We sat down to eat and try as I might Colin would not engage with me. He talked and played with Sam but blatantly ignored me. I cleared the dishes away, tidied up, put Sam to bed and tried once more. Still nothing. I was dying inside. I really couldn't believe how stubborn Colin could be. Yes, I'd seen him like this to other people, but to be like this to me, his wife, someone he lived with and purported to love. I couldn't understand how he had the energy to actively not engage with me. I felt worthless. Was I really such a horrible person to be with?

I started to question everything about myself; had I slept with the client and forgotten about it or chosen to ignore it? Had I really drunk so much the night of his birthday that I was pissed? Was I really such a bad wife? Did I really deserve to be treated like this? Was I really a bad mother? Was I wrong to be trying so hard to keep a roof over my family's head? The negative self-talk became incessant. It was never far from the surface but now it became almost deafening. I concluded that I was a bad person, an awful mother and a diabolical wife. But, I still decided to give it one last try.

I went to bed that night and vowed to try again the following morning, Saturday. As usual Colin woke me up with a cup of tea and I asked him to sit down on the bed. He did so without a word. Was this a minor breakthrough? At least, I thought, he seems to be prepared to listen now. So, I started, "I don't understand what I've done wrong and I don't understand why I'm still in the guest bedroom, we need to resolve this." He stood up and looked at me and with a sneer said.

"If you don't know what you've done wrong, you need to think about it some more," and, calling Sam, he disappeared downstairs indicating that the conversation was over and he wasn't prepared to talk about it further. But still I tried.

I got up and dressed and went downstairs into the kitchen. "Do you want a cup of tea? Bacon sandwich?" he ignored me. I decided to give him the benefit of the doubt and went into the room he was in and asked again, "Cup of tea? Bacon sandwich?" he looked at me, ignored the question and got up and walked out of the room. I knew that my attempts were futile. I made myself a cup of tea and a bacon sandwich thinking that maybe the smell of cooking bacon would encourage him to talk, but there was still nothing. Finishing my sandwich, I took my tea upstairs and started to gather up my toiletries. I packed my belongings into as many bags as possible and started loading my car. I piled my clothes and shoes into the car and took what I needed for Sam. I wasn't going to take him with me just yet as I didn't want to disrupt him, but I needed to have some of his things with me so that when I was sorted out I could set up his room and it would make his transition easier.

Colin didn't move a muscle as I was loading my car. He continued watching whatever was on TV whilst playing with our son. I finished loading my car and stood at the lounge door. Colin didn't even acknowledge my presence. "I'm going to my mother's and as soon as I'm sorted I'll be back for Sam. It's obvious to me that you don't want to be married to me any more so I'm making the decision for you. I will pick up Sam next weekend, he can spend the weekend with me." That was it, I got into my car and drove away knowing that I was leaving my second husband and ending my marriage.

I cried for the entire 30-minute drive to my parents' home. They were surprised to see me standing at their door but ushered me in as I knew they would. Sitting in their conservatory, between drinking tea and sobbing, I relayed the events of the past week or so. "What have I done wrong? What is so bad about wanting to provide for my family that I deserve to be treated like this? If there is a God, why is he doing this to me? All I've ever done is try to help people."

I was distraught, the worst thing I'd ever done was trust people too much. Unfortunately, that had been my downfall. My parents were, as ever, brilliant. They helped me unload my car and arrange their spare bedroom so that it felt homely. They made me a light lunch and then sat down and worked out an action plan.

First thing on Monday morning, whilst I was at work, they would call the local school and find out how and when Sam could start. Then they'd find details of the local letting agents and have a look to see what flats were available locally. I'd intended taking the day off from work, in fact my new job was the last thing on my mind and at this stage I really didn't care if I ever went back. It seemed to have caused me so much trouble, but my parents insisted I went to work on Monday and carried on as usual. They would do as much as they could for me and if I needed to take time off from work, then I would do so, but only if absolutely necessary. They didn't want me to lose this job knowing the situation I was in.

I went into the office on the Monday morning leaving my parents to make the necessary phone calls. As is the case in offices all over the world on a Monday morning, the question is asked of most people, "How was your weekend?" and so my client, now boss/client, asked me the same question. I gave him an appraised version of recent events and he looked thoughtful for a while before offering me a house and introducing me to his friend, a solicitor. The solicitor was one of the best divorce solicitors in Wales and he got me an appointment with her later that day. He also suggested I went and had a look at one of the houses in his property portfolio. It was a new-build property and had sat empty for the past 6-months as the recession took hold and the market for executive rental properties was in massive decline. He told me he would rather it was occupied at half the rent by someone he knew and trusted, rather than remain empty much longer. It was a beautiful house about a mile away from my parents' home so after viewing it I accepted the offer and moved in over a couple of days.

Unfortunately, the prospect of schooling Sam locally wasn't quite as straightforward and after much wrangling and protracted conversations with the local council they informed me that they didn't have a place within a 12-mile radius for Sam and I would have to wait and apply during their regular application window. Despite all of the best efforts of myself and my parents they wouldn't budge, I was left with no choice but to leave Sam with his father and collect him every Friday to spend the weekend with me, returning him on a Monday morning when I dropped him off at school. His dad wasted no time in asking me to pay maintenance and it was agreed that I would pay him £80 per week in cash. He wanted the cash so that it wouldn't impact upon his benefits. Being worn down, and unfamiliar with the benefit system, I didn't protest when my now estranged husband gave me excuse after excuse for not wanting the money to go via his bank account. I didn't have the energy to argue and he managed to make me feel guilty for leaving him to look after our son with no income. In his words I had abandoned him and Sam, he even told Sam that I'd left because I didn't love them anymore!

I didn't know at the time, but this was the way things would be for a significant number of years and putting Sam's welfare and wellbeing first in this instance was the absolute worst thing I could have done. But again, it would be some years before I discovered that.

CHAPTER 16

Things Get Worse Before They Get Better

Although leaving Colin had been my last resort, I felt very fortunate in securing a beautiful house and starting my new job. It had been heart breaking leaving Sam, but I told myself it was only for a short while until I was able to secure him a school place. Colin had started talking to me again since I had begun paying him maintenance in cash as he'd requested. Whilst our relationship wasn't brilliant, it was amicable, and we intended to keep it that way for our son. We quickly fell into an almost seamless routine of Monday to Friday with daddy, Friday evening to Monday morning with mummy. Occasionally we did things together as a family on a weekend and it seemed as if our relationship was improving. That was until I filed for divorce. I was sick of living in limbo and I wasn't prepared to spend the next however many years like this, unable to move forward with my life.

I sat with the solicitor and told her I wanted it to be quick and easy, I wanted nothing from Colin, I just wanted Sam to live with me and that was that. She advised me that I could divorce Colin on the grounds of unreasonable behaviour and it didn't take long to come up with five reasons to submit on the divorce application. All being well the divorce could be at decree nisi stage within a matter of months. Within a week I had a call from Colin, he had received the divorce petition, which he had been expecting, but he wasn't prepared to agree to the grounds of the divorce and said he wanted to divorce me instead. I couldn't see what the problem was, I told him if that was what he would prefer to do then to carry on, just write back to my solicitor stating that he was refusing the divorce petition and would be submitting a new one.

It didn't bother me, I couldn't see what grounds he could reasonably divorce me on and really didn't care, I just wanted the divorce granted so that we could both move forward with our lives.

As this rumbled on in the background so things started to become a bit strange at work. My boss, my former client, was in his mid-sixties and always fancied himself as some sort of playboy millionaire. Despite having a gorgeous second wife, he was always playing around and inevitably had some young twenty-something girl on his arm, no doubt impressed with his ability to throw his money around to try to impress people. As a client, he was pleasant enough and I could ignore his personality for the most part, but as a boss I was having to put up with his personality day in, day out. I quickly learned that the best way to handle him was to massage his ego and I decided it was easy enough to do that during office hours, I could then switch off when I returned home. Easier said than done.

Before long I was being dragged out to long lunches and then early dinners where he would take me to fancy restaurants and introduce me to the great and the good of the local business scene. It dawned on me that he was displaying me like some sort of trophy business partner. I put that thought to the back of my mind, ate lunch or dinner, never with more than one glass of wine as I was always driving, and played along.

One day in the office, he asked me if I could work on a project with him that evening. I told him I had plans but could come back at around 8pm to look at the project. He suggested meeting at his home, as it was nearer to where I was living, and not to worry about wearing business dress, just to put something comfortable on. I left the office at 5pm and arranged to meet him at 8pm at his home. When I arrived, he must have been waiting for me because the electronic gates automatically opened and he appeared at the window indicating where on the driveway I should park.

There was no sign of his wife's red Porsche, so I assumed I was being guided into a parking space that would keep room for her to return home later. I parked my car and walked to the front door where my boss opened it. I must have looked somewhat taken aback as he explained to me. "I always slip into this silk robe when I get home, it helps me relax, let me show you around."

Alarm bells started to ring in my head but I ignored them, I was just being silly, I was tense, I was tired and I was in unfamiliar surroundings. This was my boss and business partner, I was perfectly safe I told myself. My ability to work out what was reasonable and unreasonable behaviour had disappeared over the past couple of years and I really didn't trust my ability to tell right from wrong. After all, Colin had constantly told me that everything I had done, which I thought was right, was wrong. He'd found fault in all of my friends and told me that I was incapable of choosing the 'right' people to be around. It was much better if I just let him decide who we/I should spend time with and associate with. After all, 'you can't trust other people, you can only trust me, I'm the only person who really cares about what happens to you' was the paraphrase I'd become used to. So, I shrugged my concerns away and blindly followed my boss.

He started by giving me a tour of the house. I was overawed by his kitchen which he boasted, "It's just for show, why would we want to cook in it when we can eat out every night."

I was flabbergasted, as someone who loves to entertain I couldn't understand why he wasn't hosting lavish dinner parties every weekend that would spill out onto his massive manicured garden. He brushed my comments aside with. "Why? When I can afford to go out and not have anyone mess up my home?"

I had been growing more and more aware of this man's arrogance whilst I worked with him, but I really couldn't believe what I was hearing. We returned to the house and he poured me a glass of wine before offering to show me upstairs. The views from the guest bedroom were apparently incredible. which they were, and we returned downstairs to his expansive study which housed a traditional, leather inlaid desk and a leather sofa.

I sat on the sofa nursing my wine, he came and sat uncomfortably close to me. Trying to escape the discomfort I was now feeling, I asked him about the project he wanted to work on and started asking numerous inane questions. I knew that the only thing that he liked to brag about more than his conquests was his incredible ability to make money and add to the millions he already had invested.

Despite feeling uncomfortable that this man, almost my father's age, was behaving in a lecherous manner towards me, I didn't want to offend him. I could lose my job and being self-employed I wasn't sure how I would be able to go to a tribunal for sexual harassment. Besides which, I reminded myself, it's thanks to this man that I have a home and a divorce solicitor, I need to be polite.

I don't know how long I kept him talking for but I do know that he topped up my wine after each sip so that I was unable to drive home. Eventually, I think around 11pm, I told him that I needed to go to sleep and asked him to remind me where the guest bedroom was. His wife hadn't returned home but being incredibly naïve I assumed that she knew I was visiting that evening. I also assumed that she knew about me, especially as I was working with her husband. I have kicked myself many, many times for my naivety.

However, for all his arrogance and lechery he showed me to the guest bedroom and en-suite shower room and handed me some clean towels so I could use the shower the following morning. I shut the bedroom door and climbed into the bed and fell asleep until around 6.30am when I awoke in a state of confusion because I didn't recognise my surroundings. I quickly recalled the previous evening, jumped in the shower, dressed then went downstairs where my boss was drinking a cup of coffee. There was no sign of his wife. When I asked if she had arrived home safely the previous evening, he told me that she was away for a couple of days, entertaining girlfriends on their yacht.

I made my excuses, that I needed to pop home to change and have some breakfast then I would see him in the office later. I spent quite some time berating myself for putting myself in such a situation and realised that I really couldn't function on my own, that I needed Colin in order to assess situations. I jumped into the shower again when I returned to the sanctuary of my own home and cried.

How could I possibly want to divorce the man who loved me, who looked after me and who looked out for me? How could I possibly manage in the big bad world without him by my side telling me who I should and shouldn't talk to, work with or associate with? How on earth had I ever managed before I met him?

I pulled myself together, pushed my thoughts to the back of my mind and got myself dressed and into the office. As I opened the office door, the boss was holding court in the middle of the office and a silence descended. Everyone looked at me, the boss said something under his breath to a colleague, I called as cheery a 'good morning' as I could manage and disappeared into the office I shared with the boss. I logged on to my computer as the boss came in talking loudly, too loudly. "I really enjoyed your company last night. Did you enjoy the wine? It's my favourite. That power shower is incredible isn't it?"

The inane conversation more or less confirmed what I thought I already knew, but a while later as I paid a visit to the toilet, I stopped to talk to the office administrator who said to me, very quietly, "You do know he's told us all that you slept together last night and that you're an item now? He's been planning it all along." My heart sank. I started to defend myself but one look at her face told me not to bother. They were so used to his shenanigans that they would believe him over me anyway, as far as anyone in the office was concerned, I had now slept with the boss to secure my position in the business.

It hurt but I brushed it off. I needed the job and so what if people thought I'd slept with the boss? It's exactly what Colin thought anyway, so what difference did it make? I knew the truth and would just have to accept that I was tarnished by association. The nature of the job didn't help much, and it wasn't long before both the boss and I were visiting a client in London.

We were booked into a hotel and I'd ensured the administrator had booked two separate rooms. Upon arriving at the hotel, the boss checked in and came back with our room cards. I breathed a sigh of relief; until we got to the room which was on the top floor and found that they were adjoining rooms which were accessed from his side. This really wasn't helping my case at all.

However, my excitement at staying in a luxury penthouse apartment in a top hotel in London over-rode my disappointment that he was once again, trying to lure me into bed with him.

A week or so later and we had to visit another client in Portsmouth.

The boss suggested that he showed me his yacht whilst we were there as it was moored in Portsmouth marina. I'd never been aboard a privately-owned yacht before, so was more than happy to accept his invitation out of curiosity. I was sure there would be plenty of other people about. We arrived at the marina and the boss spoke to the marina manager. Then we walked along the jetty and pontoons to the yacht. It's fair to say I was impressed.

Bizarrely, we ate a salad and had a glass of wine on the yacht before returning to the car. It transpired that the boss had called ahead and said that he was taking a girlfriend to see the yacht, please could they stock the fridge with salad and wine and not disturb us for at least an hour and a half. I'm glad I didn't know that before I stepped aboard the yacht, but the knowing looks and grins as I alighted told me everything I needed to know. I most definitely wasn't the first 'girlfriend' he'd taken to his yacht and he'd inferred to everyone who knew him that he was sleeping with me. I do however, have to take responsibility for my own naivety at this time.

It didn't take long for me to start to ignore the whispers and looks from people who saw us together. I knew I wasn't sleeping with him. He could say whatever he liked. I felt sorry for him that he had to use me to boost his ego and I kept reminding myself 'sticks and stones may break my bones, but words will never hurt me'. It was difficult, but it kept me turning up at the office, smiling sweetly through gritted teeth and continuing to massage his ego. I imagined this is how hookers felt only, I figured, they were literally having sex as well. I couldn't begin to imagine how they did their job!

Inevitably it wasn't long before I was asked to work late on another project. This time I was required to stay late at the office. He took me out for dinner and we returned to the office to start working on the project, which I quickly realised was non-existent.

The project, as far as he was concerned, was to have sex with me. He'd decided as I was comfortable in the office then that would be the place it would happen, only I didn't realise it at the time as I sat down on the red leather chesterfield sofa that was in the office between both of our desks. This time he came and sat uncomfortably close and didn't even pretend that he had any other agenda.

I stood up, thanked him for dinner, told him that I couldn't possibly sleep with either my boss or a married man and made my somewhat flustered excuses. I drove home, poured myself some wine and escaped into some mindless TV until I fell asleep.

The following morning, I turned up at the office as usual, certain that he would have got over having his ego deflated, and that despite some initial awkwardness we could get on with work. How wrong I was.

Once again, he was holding court only this time he had gone into intimate detail about how we had had rampant sex on the sofa, over the desks and how I was insatiable. He'd had to promise me more sex in the office tonight, just so we could both go home and get some sleep. My eyes, heavy with the wine I had drunk at home the night before, seemed to corroborate the story and the rest of the team made up their own minds and started passing comments and jibes whenever they saw me. Laughing them off was tiring and I decided to escape the office at lunchtime and go for a walk. I had been out for around 20 minutes when my mobile rang.

It was the boss. I chose not to answer it and decided that anything he wanted could wait, I would go back after I had had a lunch hour. The phone rang at least another three times in quick succession, each time it was my boss. Again, I ignored the calls. I listened to my voicemail messages as I walked back to the office so that I knew what he was trying to get hold of me for.

"If you're not going to answer your phone when I ring it, you can forget about coming back to the office. You'll do as I tell you or you can forget about your job. Hand your keys in at the desk and don't come back you little slut." I couldn't believe it.

I had spent weeks ignoring what he had been inferring, weeks ignoring the sly glances and whispered comments of other people, and weeks trying to keep him sweet without compromising my morals and principals too much. I was exhausted by refusing his advances. I was exhausted from trying to deal with my divorce, and I was exhausted by trying to convince the outside world that everything was fine and I was happy.

I was desperately miserable, incredibly lonely, dejected, despondent, ugly, fat, unloved and only worthy of being some playboy millionaire's bit on the side. Colin had been right, he had only offered me the job for one reason, not that I was sleeping with him, but that he had expected me to sleep with him out of gratitude. That was obviously all I was good for. I should have just slept with him and accepted that it was all I was good for. Was there really anything wrong with being a high-class hooker? It was seeming like a very favourable option at this point in time.

It was with a heavy heart and a very keen awareness of the irony, I called Colin and told him that I had been sacked for refusing to sleep with the boss. It meant that I couldn't pay maintenance and I would have to work out what I would do about the house.

Colin was his unsurprising self, telling me 'it was all my fault, I had no idea what I was doing, I wasn't capable of working at that level and what was he supposed to do now that he had no income? I had ruined his life and now I was ruining my own, is that what made me happy?' Talk about hit someone when they're down.

I was well and truly on my own and had no idea what I was going to do. I needed to think, I needed to take action but most of all I needed help, fast!

CHAPTER 17

Maybe This Time?

Whenever I've gone through the upset and despair of bad news, or an upsetting event, I have an incredible ability to become very resourceful and do *whatever it takes*. So, having been royally sacked, I drowned my sorrows for an evening or two, then did what my parents had done for me previously, I worked out an action plan. First things first, I needed an income. I decided to call the benefits office, the dole office, call them what you will.

I had never applied for benefits before and truly believed that as I had paid in for all of my working life, I could tell them what had happened over recent months and they would tell me how much I could claim in benefits to help me when I needed it most. I can honestly say it was the most degrading, soul-destroying, humiliating situation I have ever been in, bar none, in my entire life. I will never, ever, go back to that again regardless of whatever dire straits I might find myself in. I'd rather live in a cardboard box than face that judgement and humiliation ever again.

Which is exactly what I said to them. After 3 weeks of being questioned, judged, being told I wasn't trying hard enough to find work, being told I didn't qualify for any benefits because I'd been self-employed and being told that I wasn't entitled to anything because I wasn't a single parent with a child living with me. Had I been a stereotypical single mother, that is, had Sam been living with me instead of his father, I would have had money thrown at me hand over fist and been given help with housing. Because I was on my own and with no resident child I was eligible for approximately £26 per week which would be paid directly into my back account.

I couldn't have help with housing and I wasn't entitled to anything else anyway because I was an undischarged bankrupt. I had always believed that by being an honest, hard-working citizen, I would have access to the help I needed should there ever come a time when I was unfortunate enough to require it. That time was now.

Whilst everything was going on with my client, I had taken the tough decision to file for personal bankruptcy. I had weighed everything up and realised that it was, by far, the best option and would alleviate some of the pressure and stress on me. My credit-rating was significantly damaged by putting the business into administration and it would take about 6 years to improve that. A bankruptcy sits on your file for 6 years, so I decided that it was the best option. I sought advice before going down that route, and subsequently on 7 July 2011 I became bankruptcy number 519 in the local County Court after paying the £500 in cash it then cost to declare yourself bankrupt and answering a number of questions from the judge.

I left the court in bright sunshine and walked along the road to where my car was parked convinced I had a flashing neon sign above my head proclaiming 'Failure' in bright pink letters with an arrow pointing down at me. It took many years for me to realise that bankruptcy was not a badge I was wearing for all to see, but the shame and failure I felt as a result of it might as well have been tattooed on my forehead. As far as I was concerned I'd let everyone down and I was an embarrassment to my family and friends. Despite now knowing that this wasn't the case, I can't change how I felt at the time and that feeling seemed to pervade every aspect of my life.

Now, not only was I bankrupt and with a failed business behind me, I was heading for my second divorce, which was still rumbling around in the background., I had lost a job I had secured simply because the person offering me the job assumed I was desperate enough to sleep with them to maintain some security. As if that wasn't enough, the benefits department were treating me as if I was the lowest of the low and insisting that I attended job seekers sessions where I would be taught how to apply for a job, write an application letter and create a CV. It didn't help that the clerk telling me all of this was fresh out of school and when asked what salary I was looking for and hearing my response, responded with, "That's three times what I earn, I don't think we get any jobs for that amount in here."

I politely told him that I would find my own job, I knew how to write a letter, I had a strong CV and that when they could introduce me to someone in senior management who could help me secure a job in the salary bracket I was looking for and worthy of I would return. But, I pointed out, until that time I would not be asking potential employers, who I was meeting for informal chats over a cup of coffee, if they would sign my job-seekers manual to prove I was actually looking for work!

The benefits agency seemed surprised that I was motivated enough to want to find work. Like I said, it was the most depressing situation I have ever been in, and if I am unfortunate enough to find myself in a similar situation again I will do anything rather than apply for benefits. I recall writing a letter to David Cameron, the then Prime Minister, saying much the same thing and some months later receiving a letter back from one of his minions suggesting I contact the Citizens Advice Bureau with help in applying for benefits. That letter ended up in the bin!

I did what I had done when I started my business, I got on the telephone. One of the people I called was the managing director of the company I had left to start my business. The company had been sold to a much larger organisation leaving all of the directors incredibly wealthy and worth a few million pounds. The Chairman and Chief Executive, who I'd worked directly for, had been let go but most of the other staff remained. That included the managing director who was now the Business Development Director for the region. He and I had kept in touch and he suggested I went to see him in his office for a chat over a cup of coffee.

A couple of days later I turned up, drank coffee and he offered me a job if I was prepared to commute from my home town to the next largest city. I would become the Business Development Manager for the company in that area. It came with the salary I was looking for and a company car. I had no problem in getting up early enough to travel the 30 or so miles to be in the office by 8.30am each day. He even agreed that I could work in my local office on a Friday so that I wasn't caught up in the usual Friday traffic. All that needed to happen was for me to meet his boss, the Regional Director, to get his approval.

We met a couple of days later and before I knew it, an offer letter was in my hands and I started my new job. The relief and security I felt at working once again for a global organisation was palpable, I started to relax once more. I was able to start paying maintenance (in cash again) to my estranged husband. I was handing over a significant amount of money to my bankruptcy trustees to enable them to repay my debts and I was starting to build something resembling a social life. I even started dating again. Not that Sam or Colin ever knew about it, but I started to feel alive once more. Things could work out.

One Monday afternoon when I was at home having taken a couple of days off work, I was pottering around the house when I heard a car drive along the gravel driveway towards the house. I wasn't particularly in the mood for visitors, so I hid. This meant that I couldn't be seen through the floor to ceiling windows, but I could still see who was driving up my drive.

A large white Range Rover appeared and a lady got out. It was my divorce solicitor. She approached the front door and I answered it. Rather than her usual welcoming demeanour, she thrust a letter into my hands and told me that she was no longer acting for me as she was now acting on behalf of her friend (the man who had sacked me for not having sex with him).

The letter was 'notice to quit' his house as he didn't want me living there anymore. The penny dropped; he had offered me the house as he thought it would be a nice little love-shack where he could visit me as the mood took him. I would be so grateful to him for giving me a job and a home that I would submit to whatever he asked of me, whenever he asked. A nice little bolt-hole where his wife wouldn't find him.

This also further suggested to me that the rumours about my solicitor and him were true. Apparently she was madly in love with him and wanted him to herself. However, he refused to become romantically involved with her, which drove her mad. She would do whatever he asked of her just to prove to him that she loved him. It was wrong, it was perverse and it was true.

I felt like I was in the middle of a really bad soap opera.

I thanked her for the letter and assured her she would have my response within a day or two. I then proceeded to report my former boss to the now non-existent Financial Services

Authority and her to the Law Society. I have no idea of the outcome of my complaints, I have no wish to know and I really don't care. I do know that the former boss lost his business some years later and lost at least half of his fortune to his second wife when she divorced him for every last penny she could get. Of the solicitor, I have no idea what happened. I believe the practice she started and built up is still trading, but I understand that she no-longer practices. Again, I don't care and have no desire to find out.

Whatever happened, happened and if my complaints against them played a part in that then so be it. If they didn't, then they were served by karma and for that I'm grateful. I then found myself another divorce solicitor and whilst my complaints were being investigated, I decided I would become a sitting tenant and refuse to pay a single penny more of rent. I had gone through so much in the past 6 months there was no way I was going to be bullied or harassed by Tweedle-Dum and Tweedle-Dee (as I had named the ex-boss and my now ex-solicitor).

A sure sign of their arrogance was their complete incomprehension that I would possibly dare to take action. They started to pay unexpected visits to the house in a bid to intimidate me. They were never physically intimidating, but they would turn up and let me know they were there and that I was breaking the law by remaining in the property and not paying rent. I have to be honest, I arrived home each evening wondering whether or not I would be able to get into the house and was always somewhat relieved when the key turned in the lock. A couple of weeks of this and I'd had enough, I called the police and reported them for intimidation and harassment and asked the police to visit them, citing tenancy law, that I had a right to live in peace and undisturbed. Whether the police visited them or not I really don't know but I didn't have any further visits from them.

My situation however, was taking its toll not just on me but on my parents too. My mother pleaded with me to give up the house and move back in with them. I resisted for as long as I could because this made me feel like a failure once more, but I couldn't stand the guilt I felt at the amount of stress my mother was under.

It was affecting my father as well, although he wouldn't show it as openly as my mother would. Still fearful of uprooting Sam again, I promised my parents I would consider it. The next weekend, after picking Sam up, I asked him how he would like it if I went and lived with Nanny and Grampy instead of staying in the big house we were in. At now 4 years old, I wasn't really expecting him to have an opinion, but I wanted to try to work out how he would handle it. All he could see was the extra spoiling he would have, more ice-cream than mum let him eat, more sweeties, more cakes, more cuddles and more time with Nanny and Grampy. It was a win-win for a 4 year old boy!

I visited my parents and told them I would move in by the end of the month and would stay with them for no more than a year. I was 38 years old and I couldn't keep running back and forth to my parents' home every time something went wrong. I needed to stand on my own two feet. Over the course of the next two weeks I gradually moved all my belongings, except for the large items, to my parents' home. Then I booked a man with a van, a friend of my father, to collect my larger items – bed, wardrobe, sofa. My parents, who only live in a traditional 3-bed semi-detached house, cleared their middle room so that I would have my own lounge and cleared their guest bedroom so that I could move in. Their box-room became Sam's weekend bedroom and any surplus furniture went into storage, until such time as I would need it again. I didn't tell my landlord that I was moving out of the property, I let him find that out for himself when his solicitors' letters remained unanswered and the rent remained unpaid. I didn't care about him. I wasn't going to lose any sleep over my behaviour towards him or any inconvenience my action might cause him or his solicitor. However, this behaviour on my part was totally at odds with how I would normally behave.

I'm someone who is very fair, often too lenient, preferring to give people the benefit of the doubt until I'm given good reason not to. I've since learned if I'm given a good reason not to be fair with someone, or to give them that benefit of the doubt, then I can be a very, very tough opponent and will do *whatever it takes* to stand up for myself, Sam, our rights and those of my family. I can be a tough cookie when I want to be!

Finally, I had a good job, I was living with my parents where I could have time to de-stress from the past few months and I could be looked after. My father had been a chef before he retired, and he loved having his eldest daughter at home. My dinner was on the table every night when I arrived home. I had to remember to call him or let him know the day before if I was going to be late or eating out with friends. I was thoroughly spoiled, I felt my strength and energy returning. It was never going to be easy living with my parents after years of living alone or married, but we made it work.

We became good friends and somehow managed to find the balance between giving each other space and spending time together. That's not to say it wasn't without its arguments or disagreements, but for the most part we all got along really well and had, and still have, a great relationship. If I could change anything, it would be that I hadn't put my parents through so much stress for most of my adult life. Thankfully, they've never held it against me and we continue to have a great relationship.

It was difficult moving back in with my parents at almost 40 years of age, I often felt like I was a failure and a disappointment to them. They never made me feel that way, but that was what the voice in my head was telling me. I was more determined than ever to do *whatever it takes* to ensure

I moved out within a year. I knew I could work to deadlines. I was going to use this as an opportunity to take back control of my life and build a stronger future.

CHAPTER 18

History Repeating

Life was going well, I was enjoying my job and getting on well with colleagues, my year of being an undischarged bankrupt was flying by and I was slowly developing a social life. I was seeing Sam every weekend and I was going on occasional dates during the week. I still wasn't divorced, but I could start to see a future.

I arrived at the office one Monday morning to be told that there was going to be a staff meeting later that day and I needed to rearrange my last appointment so that I could be there. My heart sank. This sounded ominous. I had arranged enough staff meetings as a PA to know that when staff were being called together with little notice and being told to rearrange appointments so that they could be there, the news generally wasn't good. I was right.

The company was restructuring and merging, which meant there would be duplicates of some jobs. In the new company they wouldn't need two of each role so the majority of us were put through consultation and put on notice of possible redundancy. I didn't need anyone to spell it out for me. I had gone into the company when their reputation was lower than low, I had worked hard at rebuilding bridges, but it hadn't, as yet, generated any actual work, just promises of work when the industry picked up.

This was construction, we were in the middle of what would be the worst recession for decades and no-one was building. I knew, just knew, that I was going to be made redundant within weeks.

I didn't wait to be told. I rearranged my diary so that I was doing the absolute minimum I needed to do in order not to find myself on the end of a disciplinary hearing before being made redundant and I spent the rest of my time sat in the office job-hunting.

There wasn't much around for a relatively inexperienced Business Development Manager in the construction industry, and I had some fun finding some dubious sounding jobs on random websites and boosting morale in our small office by allocating these strange occupations to members of the team.

I decided we could all form a co-operative, take these abstruse jobs and then all write the stories that would undoubtedly arise from such obscure roles. It caused much hilarity amongst us all, and my last days in that office will always be remembered fondly and with joy.

Amongst these mysterious jobs, I did manage to find a very small lineage advert requesting a business development manager for a facilities management company back in my home town.

The salary was only slightly less than I was currently on and it came with a company car. I submitted my CV and covering email. Less than three hours later, I received a telephone call inviting me for interview, which I subsequently arranged for the Friday of that week when I would be based in the company office in my home town.

Ironically it would be the same day that I was issued with a formal redundancy notice for a number of weeks' time.

The managing director was upset when he handed me my redundancy letter. There were tears in his eyes when he said to me, "If I'd known this was on the cards so soon I would never have offered you the position, you've been through enough, you don't need this as well." I was surprisingly circumspect, dignified and calm as I responded to him and said, "It's no surprise, I was the last one in. I'm the least experienced BDM in the company it's just business. I know that you haven't hand-picked me as the person that has to go. It doesn't make sound business sense to keep me on. You gave me the chance and opportunity when I desperately needed one and I will always be grateful for that."

And it's true, I will always be grateful for that, but it didn't stop me sobbing later that evening and asking anyone who would listen, "Why can't I get a job? Why will no-one employ me? I want to work, I'm capable of working, why will no-one take me on as a PA?" I had been rejected for more PA jobs than I could remember, so I now had to continue to try to find business development roles to build up my experience on my CV.

I'd had my interview with this new company and I was waiting to hear from them. As if in answer to my questions my mobile rang. I didn't recognise the number so answered it thinking it might be one of the directors who had interviewed me earlier, letting me down gently.

I was right, it was one of the directors from my earlier interview but instead of letting me down, they were offering me the job. I accepted, ended the conversation then sat down and cried some more. Maybe, just maybe, there was someone 'up there' looking out for me after all.

All I had to do now was wait for my job offer to arrive, then I could let my soon to be former employer know when I would be leaving. I hadn't been there long enough to qualify for a redundancy payment so, as far as I was concerned, it was about staying long enough just to hand over to the person who would be taking on my role as well as their own and tying up any loose ends. I worked just one more week for them.

CHAPTER 19

Third Time Lucky

The following Monday I had something of a lie in, not having to commute 30 miles to the office, and drove the five miles to my new place of work. Within a few hours they had asked me to assist with internal business development. I was asked to write a report at the end of my first month identifying areas where they could make improvements in business efficiency, improved processes and cost savings. They also wanted me to get out and about making myself known to existing clients. The first month was a whirl of activity.

They were a fast-growing business. I was quickly introduced by one director or another to all of the clients and I started to get a good understanding of the business. I was still living with my parents, working through my bankruptcy, seeing Sam every weekend, paying maintenance in cash, building a social life and looking to the future.

On the surface everything seemed great, but something wasn't right. I couldn't put my finger on it, but I wasn't comfortable working for this new company. I put it down to nerves and my self-doubt returning. There seemed to be a strange atmosphere in the company and I couldn't work out what it was. I ignored my niggles and carried on regardless; I was sure whatever it was would sort itself out eventually.

At the end of my first month I submitted my report to the directors as I had been asked. Amongst my recommendations I said that they needed to deploy or dismiss their administrator and PA. Neither of them were experienced and weren't capable of the jobs they were being paid to do. I told them that I would not have employed either of them in my PA business, they just weren't good enough. I also asked them why they had employed me. It was evident that they couldn't afford my position and they did much better business development themselves. I was very much a spare part they would be better off without.

They dismissed that recommendation and chose to ignore my comments about the PA and administrator. I soon learned why – the PA and administrator were both sleeping with the same director!

Over the next few months I noticed some distinct animosity between the two directors. The quieter, but more genuine of the two, appeared more and more withdrawn and was spending less and less time in the office. The other was displaying more peacock-type behaviour, becoming more and more arrogant and it was quite frankly unpleasant to be associated with him.

Once again, I started to do just the bare minimum I could get away with and began to look around for another job. I didn't know what was going on in the company, but the feeling I'd had when I started, that something wasn't right, was still there and was becoming more urgent with each passing day. Something was going to erupt before long and I didn't think it would be pleasant.

I'd developed quite a good relationship with the other three managers in the company. I started to ask them about the directors and tentatively broached the subject of this 'feeling' I'd been having. Two of them didn't want to talk about it and told me that whilst they weren't happy in their roles they couldn't move. They wouldn't expand any further on why, in fact they seemed to clam up. They weren't happy but refused to do anything about it. Rather than saying that they didn't want to, or giving some excuse why they couldn't or why they stayed put, they just said that they couldn't move and that's all there was to it. I found their attitude strange, I'd never come across it before.

The other manager on the other hand loved to talk. He was often teased for taking half an hour to explain something when it should only have taken 10 minutes. Because I would listen to him, he was often sent by the others to talk to me, or they would wander over and include me in their conversations with him so that they could make their exit. I decided I would ask him about my 'feeling'.

Not being completely familiar with his area of the business I suggested that he and I went out to the local coffee shop so that he could tell me about the section he managed and fill me in on how his department fitted in with all of the others. We arranged to meet, told everyone where we were going and went for a coffee.

After talking about his department, I asked him about the company ethos and culture. I instinctively knew that this feeling of mine was about the ethos and culture so that seemed as good a place as any to start.

I recall him looking at me as if he was a rabbit caught in the headlights, sucking in a deep breath between pursed lips then telling me what he knew or what he had heard. It didn't make for good listening and I knew that I was doing the right thing in looking for a different job.

He confided in me that he was also planning his exit but keeping it quiet until the time was right. I promised to help him where I could with any contacts I had. He was hoping to start his own business, not in competition with our employer but certainly within the same field.

The atmosphere within the company was one of fear, intimidation and blatant sexism. Whilst I had noticed the sexism instantly it was the fear and intimidation that I had picked up on but not identified. Within minutes of my colleague sharing his first-hand experience I knew that I had to get out.

The senior director thought he was some kind of Mafioso Godfather who really did instill fear into anyone who had the audacity to disagree with him or suggest that there was a better way of doing things. My colleague was terrified that his plans would be discovered before he left the company. He pleaded with me not to say anything. I assured him of my discretion and kept my word.

Some weeks later I was summoned into the office, the meeting started with them complaining about my use of social media in my own time. They didn't like me saying I wasn't happy in my job, even though I never mentioned the company name and didn't link to people who I worked with.

They had been following my Twitter feed (I'd discovered and embraced both Twitter and Facebook by this time) and even complained that I was posting too late at night or too early in the morning. I told them I had insomnia. I couldn't be bothered to explain to them that I pre-scheduled some posts because I was just maintaining a profile for when I became self-employed again and besides, what I chose to do in my own time was none of their business. It certainly had nothing to do with them whether I slept or not. I wasn't damaging their profile, I wasn't naming them and I wasn't saying what work I was doing. They were getting paranoid.

Later the same day, I was asked to find some information on my computer. I went straight to the file where the document had been stored to find it was missing. Another summons to the office, this time to be hauled over the coals for stealing files that belonged to them.

I knew I hadn't stolen any files. There was nothing about the company I would want to steal for myself or anyone else. I also knew that this was one of the tactics they had used to dismiss the person who had previously had my role, my colleague had warned me of that.

I really couldn't be bothered to argue and suggested there and then that as they were obviously unhappy with me I should leave with immediate effect, and that's what happened. I went out of the office, collected my personal belongings and left, calling cheery goodbyes to my colleagues as I left. I was free. Free from the joke that was that business.

Some months later, I learned that the second director had been forcibly bought out of the business. My former colleague, who had left and started his own business, had had to move to a new town and establish a new identity to protect himself and his family after being threatened by men in balaclavas and wielding baseball bats in his own home; sent at the behest of our former employer.

Unfortunately, he was unable to bring charges as no-one would stand as a witness.

Thankfully that colleague and his family are now very happy and very safe.

I was back to square one, no job, no income and living with my parents.

And I was still an undischarged bankrupt!

Thankfully, during the 3 years of growing my business I had developed a really good network of contacts. One of them had heard of my situation and gave me a call out of the blue and asked to meet for coffee. He then asked if I'd join his company as a Business Consultant. In his words, "Your experience is worth far more to me than someone with a certificate who's just read about it."

I joined his company on a year-long contract and thoroughly enjoyed my time working there. I was setting up businesses on behalf of my client, taking them through incubation, testing their feasibility and if they proved feasible passing them on to someone else to head up and develop further. If they weren't likely to go anywhere, then they got shelved.

I was in my element and felt as if life was starting to take a turn for the better, and it certainly was. It wasn't long before I was able to move out of my parents' home and rent my own flat in a dream location on top of a cliff.

My flat, well technically it was a maisonette as it was over two floors, was on the top of a cliff about 10 metres from the edge with nothing to spoil my view. I had floor to ceiling picture windows in my bedroom and lounge and Sam had his own massive bedroom which had more than enough space for his bed and for him to play and leave toys out all over the place if he wanted to. I couldn't have been happier.

Unfortunately, my parents had to act as rent guarantors due to my bankruptcy, but I assured them they had no reason to worry as I wasn't going to calling upon them. I knew that if I defaulted on my rent it would cost my parents a significant amount of their pensions and I wasn't going to let that happen, particularly after all they had done for me.

Life was on the up, I had a regular income and I felt secure in my position. They say that pride comes before a fall and whilst I was quietly celebrating my new-found good fortune, I forgot that I was on a contract with a finite time and so forgot to build up my own business in the background. You might well ask, "How on earth could you forget?" Given what I'd been through, the sheer relief and excitement of having a regular income and doing a job I enjoyed and in which I felt valued lulled me into a somewhat false sense of security. It also taught me a valuable lesson.

The day the contract ended came as a bit of a shock but at the same time whilst unprepared for it, I wasn't surprised. It was all completely above board and I was still asked to do some ad-hoc work, but that wasn't quite as secure as I'd become used to.

I think in my own little world, I had told myself that they would be so happy with the good job I was doing that they wouldn't want me to go and they'd extend the contract. I recognise now that that was a way of me not facing up to my fears of not being able to hold down a job or being capable of getting a job. I was also scared of the unknown 'what if' that might mean I couldn't afford to pay for my beautiful flat. The day after my contract ended I sat and cried with despair, fear and self-loathing. My self-talk continued, "How could I have been so stupid as to not think ahead? Why didn't I build my business quietly in the background? How on earth was I going to pay next month's rent?"

What the f*!k was I going to do now?

I tried my best not to panic and did all I could to rein in any unnecessary spending, which wasn't an easy task given that I was still paying a significant sum to the trustees of my bankruptcy! I cut back on my food shopping, buying a chicken or small joint of meat each week and cooking a roast dinner with loads of veg then making that last all week by being inventive with leftover meat and vegetables.

I started foraging to make blackberry crumbles for dessert for me and Sam, making the foraging trip part of a Saturday afternoon or Sunday morning adventure. I learned to eat (and enjoy) porridge for breakfast and I discovered the value/basic brands of my local supermarket. I put less petrol into my car and walked more and found some new enthusiasm for getting on my 'clapped out' bicycle. I stopped buying newspapers and magazines, stopped having coffee and cake when I met friends, choosing to drink water and not eat instead. I changed my mobile phone contract and I started using freecycle.com and other buy/sell/swap sites when I wanted or needed something new instead of just giving things away to them as I had done before.

I started to dye my own hair and just decided to grow it even longer rather than visit the hairdresser. I bought cheap/own brand skin care and cosmetics rather than my usual luxury brands. It was difficult to cut back on utility bills as I didn't use much in the way of gas and electricity anyway. I cut back on as much as I possibly could because I wasn't prepared to cut back on Sam's weekend drama and dance clubs. He loved his clubs and had started them as soon as he was old enough, having attended numerous rehearsals with me over the years and asking, "When can I go on stage like you mummy?" I'd told him he needed to learn to read properly first (so that he could sight-read scripts) and then promised him I'd find him a class he could attend on a Saturday. That was my absolute non-negotiable and remains the same today.

Those cutbacks bought me a month or two of extra money and gave me some time to find more work. I updated my CV and sent it out with a covering letter to every administrative/PA/secretarial job that was advertised in my area. I didn't receive a single invitation to interview and only a handful of 'thanks but no thanks' letters.

Many were from people I knew, people who knew I was more than capable of doing the job I was applying for. When I called to ask for feedback as to why I was unsuccessful, of those who had the courtesy to talk to me or respond by email, they all said the same thing, "You're over qualified, we know you can do the job with your eyes shut but you've been self-employed for a couple of years, you'll get bored here and leave. Then we'll have to recruit again."

I often responded with, "Why don't you let me decide whether I'll get bored and leave? Why don't you believe that I actually want the stability of a normal job with a regular wage?" But my protestations got me nowhere.

Four months after my fixed-term contract ended I was unemployed and seemingly unemployable.

I struggled with accepting my situation. I couldn't believe I had let myself get into this position and I knew I faced the very real prospect of losing my home and possibly declaring bankruptcy for a second time within a year. Was it even possible to declare bankruptcy again when you were only just discharged from your first bankruptcy? I didn't know, and I didn't want to find out.

How was I going to tell my parents that my promises that they wouldn't have to bail me out as guarantors for my rent were going to have to be reneged upon?

I was 39 years old and an abject failure. What was wrong with me? Why couldn't I just do things right? Why did it seem so easy for everyone else to have a normal life but so difficult for me?

I couldn't understand what I'd done wrong. All I'd ever wanted, all I'd ever tried to do, was to create a loving family home. I was honest almost to a fault, I never lied, cheated or stole. I was polite and knew my manners and always treated others as I wanted them to treat me. In short, I was properly brought up, I'd always behaved myself and done as I was told yet somehow it wasn't enough.

Was it wrong to have a little bit of ambition and want the best for me and my family? If it was, how did so many other people manage to achieve it?

I decided that it was my fault. That I was, as Colin had told me, incapable of running a business and had no right to think I was. I was obviously a diabolical mother otherwise Sam would have been living with me. It was blatantly apparent to anyone that I was a rubbish PA because otherwise I'd have a job by now.

It became clear to me that all of the people who had been friends with me were only my friends because I'd had a relatively high profile in the local area. My star had been on the ascendency, they obviously only wanted to come along for the ride. Colin had told me often enough that people didn't like me, well, I reasoned with myself, he was right.

It's fair to say that during this period my self-esteem, self-confidence and self-worth were well into negative figures. I'd started to self-medicate with alcohol and as Lisa Nicholson says in her book "No Matter What!", I was 'looking for love through a door marked sex'. This only served to make me feel even worse about myself when I sobered up the following day. I'd be fine for a couple of days, then drown my sorrows again, look for love through the door marked sex, and so the vicious circle would start again. I hated myself and couldn't see how anyone else could possibly like me, let alone love me.

It was time to take responsibility, be a big girl and do everyone a favour and so I came up with a plan. Over the next few days I visited various shops to buy what I needed. I didn't need much but I couldn't buy all that I wanted in just one shop, my bulk purchase would be queried. I didn't want anyone to have any idea of what I was planning. It didn't take me long to drain the bottle of wine that I had bought for this purpose and then I opened the vodka, which I'd also purchased for this very purpose. I took a sip to get used to the taste, it was sharp and caused me to draw in breath between my teeth in the way you see actors do in films when they're drowning their sorrows. I was putting all of my hopes in this magical liquid and the piles of what looked like sweets that were now sitting on my desk.

My requests to the Universe, to God or whoever/whatever were listening to include me in a fatal accident hadn't come to fruition, it was time to take matters into my own hands.

The taste of the vodka was sharp against my tongue, but it felt good. I knew this was going to work. I picked up the first pile of mixed pills in my left hand, I had no idea what was there altogether but I didn't care. There was a mix of old prescription drugs for ailments long since forgotten and whatever I'd been able to purchase over-the-counter.

And so, we're back to where this book began; these unassuming white disks and ovals had a job to do. I reached for the vodka with my right hand and tipped my head back to pour the pills into my mouth. It was then that I caught sight of the photograph of Sam. It brought me to my senses quicker than someone slapping my face would have done. I realised I couldn't do this to Sam. There had to be another way. Sobbing I cleared away the paraphernalia I'd collected to execute my plan and allowed my frustration, anger, hopelessness and desolation to come flooding through me.

"Better out than in." I thought, recalling the words my parents would say to me when I was sick as a child. How ironic that it would be my parents' words that calmed me down at this precise moment when I'd planned to save them the embarrassment and disappointment of having to look after their eldest daughter again.

Tired from crying, but strangely lucid, I poured my magical elixir down the sink and flushed the sweetie-pills down the toilet. I had to find another way. "There's always a solution," again my parents' words entered my head. No matter what I did, I would save them questioning themselves if I wasn't here. I knew my parents well enough and knew that they would blame themselves had I succeeded in my original plan. They would have asked why I hadn't talked to them, asked why I felt I couldn't go back to them. I realised that this would have caused them far more pain and distress than me removing myself from the situation. I had to sit down, take stock and look at what I had that could earn me some money.

In my somewhat inebriated state, I was forming the basis of a fairly coherent but frightening plan. I had no idea how it was going to work, I had no idea what I was going to do but I had to start somewhere. I was prepared to do *whatever it took* to create change and so I sent a text message to a friend of mine.

"What's the name of that website you told me about?"

She responded almost instantly, as I knew she would and asked. "Are you alright hun?"

"Yes," I responded. "I'll call you in the morning."

Now that I knew where to start I had intense clarity and I had work to do. If I didn't start to take action straight away I'd talk myself out of this crazy, ludicrous idea by the time I'd slept on it.

When I fell into an alcohol, tear and fear-induced coma a couple of hours later I had a business homepage. Within 24-hours I had my first client. This was to be a short-lived business venture, but it gave me enough time to put my finances in order, put myself back onto an even keel and find myself a long-term temporary position. It taught me many, many things about myself, more about human-kind than I ever thought I'd learn, changed many preconceptions and judgements and surprisingly altered my view of the world for the better.

But one thing was certain, I would never be the same again and the term 'whatever it takes' would take on a completely different meaning but that's a story for another day.

CHAPTER 21

Act 1 - Epilogue - The Here and Now

Fast forward a couple of years and I'm in a very different place. Somehow or other I found the strength to carry on. My mantra had been *whatever it takes*. My strength came from constantly telling myself that I was going through all of this so that no-one else had to.

Having decided that life certainly was worth living, I vowed to one day write about my story. I decided that if it could help just one other person feel less lonely or give them strength to keep going through whatever they're going through, then my adventures through adversity will have been worth it.

First of all, I had to work out how to rebuild my life. It wasn't easy but I knew I needed to do it for me and for Sam, and I had to make it so much better than it had ever been before.

I now live my life on my terms. Sam lives with me and attends a local school. He has a busy active social life as you would expect of any teenager and spends some time with his dad. We live near the coast with the love of my life whom I first met 20 years ago and reconnected with whilst realising a lifelong ambition in 2013.

Life's funny like that, you hit major lows and you'll know that. For a long time I thought that was how my life was meant to be, but as soon as I decided I was going to start living on my terms, or as I like to say, I stepped out of the wings into my spotlight, life changed and all of a sudden, I was and am living it in full technicolour.

If you'd like to know more about how my life changed and how you too can Step Out of the Wings Into YOUR Spotlight please look out for my next book "Create Your Blockbuster Life: Step Out of the Wings Into YOUR Spotlight" where I share the hints, tips and strategies I put into place to create my own blockbuster life. I won't tell you what you should be doing or how you should be living, I simply share what I know works to enable you to live YOUR life on YOUR terms.

It's time for you to produce your own blockbuster, for you to step out of the wings into your spotlight and to rewrite your script and shine.

Thank you so much for reading my story, I hope it has helped or inspired you in some way. If you wish to find out more, or would like to share your story or how you have stepped out of the wings into your spotlight, please get in touch here.

www.notarehearsal.co.uk

notarehearsal@outlook.com

Shine bright

Deborah-Jane

Where to Get Help

I couldn't finish a book like this without offering some kind of help, support of guidance. Whilst *'Whatever it Takes'* is very much my story, and all stories are different, it would be irresponsible of me not to offer some sort of help or assistance.

I sincerely hope that you picked up this book because you are interested in real-life stories of ordinary people but there is also a very strong likelihood that you picked this book up because a part of it resonated with you. If that is the case I would like to share with you the Cycle of Abuse which was shared with me as I was coming to the realisation that I had been in an abusive relationship.

I am relating this to a psychologically abusive relationship but you will see from it that it applies to physically abusive relationships too.

The Cycle of Abuse

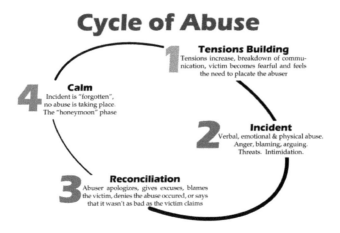

Cycle of Abuse

1 Tensions Building
Tensions increase, breakdown of communication, victim becomes fearful and feels the need to placate the abuser

2 Incident
Verbal, emotional & physical abuse. Anger, blaming, arguing. Threats. Intimidation.

3 Reconciliation
Abuser apologizes, gives excuses, blames the victim, denies the abuse occured, or says that it wasn't as bad as the victim claims

4 Calm
Incident is "forgotten", no abuse is taking place. The "honeymoon" phase

Cycle of Abuse image: © http://violentrelationships.blogspot.com/

1.   Tensions Building

This is the stage where you know something's wrong. You probably don't know what but you are noticing those warning signs that your partner isn't happy. You're probably walking on egg-shells and desperately trying to make sure you do the right thing, whatever that might be. The likelihood is that even the right thing will be the wrong thing for your partner. You probably feel quite nervous and tense.

2.   Incident

In the relationship you're in this might be an argument, it could be your partner deciding they or you are not going to attend an event you've been looking forward to because of something you've supposedly done. Their insults and threats will increase and they will probably start blaming all sorts of things on you. This will be the flash-point where you are left in no doubt that you've done something seriously wrong in the eyes of your partner.

3.   Reconciliation

You'll receive an apology, either directly or it will be something really subtle that you'll recognise is your partner's apology. They'll excuse the incident, blaming it on someone or something else. You might even be told it was your fault. Alternatively, they'll make you believe that the incident wasn't as bad as you think it was. However, they colour it, you will be left under no illusion that as far as they're concerned the incident is over and forgotten.

4.   Calm

Life carries on as normal, as if nothing has happened. Your partner will be treating you with grace and respect and you'll probably be wondering if you imagined everything to do with the incident. This will continue until the next time tensions start to build and the cycle will start again.

There is no fixed time-scale for each phase of this cycle. Every relationship is different and for some people this cycle will go from stage 1 to 4 in the course of day, for others it will occur over the course of days, weeks or even months. However long it takes, you will undoubtedly recognise the cycle.

I would also like to share with you the text of the bookmark that was included with this book.

These bookmarks are distributed in public places and schools. They have been very effective in highlighting to teenagers the features of a healthy relationship and when they should pay attention to warning signs. The text is reproduced here so you always have it should your bookmark get lost or damaged.

Loves Me	Loves Me Not
Signs of a loving relationship	Tries to control me
Makes me feel safe	Gets violent, loses temper quickly
Makes me feel comfortable	Always blame me
Listens to me	Is sexually demanding
Values my opinions	Keeps me from seeing my friends and family
Supports what I want to do in life	Makes all the decisions
Is truthful with me	Embarrasses me in front of others
Always tries to understand how I feel	Hits me
Likes that I have other friends	Makes me cry
Makes me laugh	Makes me feel afraid
Trusts me	Is always 'checking up' on me
Treats me as an equal	Takes my money and other things
Respects my family	Threatens to leave me if do not do as I am told
Understands my need for time alone or with family	Teases, bullies and puts me down
Accepts me as I am	

www.soroptimist-gbi.org

© Soroptimist International Yeovil & District

140

If you recognise any of these signs you may be a victim of abuse. You DO NOT have to suffer alone.

National Domestic Abuse Freefone Helpline: 0808 2000 247

Childline: 0800 1111

Somerset DAFFS: 0800 694 9999

All relationships go through difficult patches but a normal healthy relationship will spend more time in the Calm stage than in any other stage.

If you have any concerns at all about your relationship please contact one of the organisations listed on the next pages.

Websites you can visit:

www.refuge.org.uk
www.womensaid.org.uk

Acknowledgements

I am eternally grateful for the people in my life who have been there for me throughout my time in the wings and in the spotlight;

- mum and dad, who in 50 years of marriage have been by my side constantly.
- My sister for no-nonsense straight talking, prosecco and camping.
- My partner, Alun, who always believed in me even when we weren't together and is my rock, sounding board and soul mate.
- Julie London, Julie Japan, Gel and Sandy all too far away but for being '3am friends'... and people too numerous to mention who supported my various business ventures one way or another.

To my legal team who have always believed in me; Wayne, Melanie, Judge Price – Thank you.

To my Open University team for increasing my understanding and confidence; Fred, Ana, Julie and Kaye.

To Yvette, Clare T-M, Tamsen, Paula, Russ, Tara for reading drafts, providing feedback and being brutally honest but equally gentle with me.

To Ann, my publisher, who has known for years that I was writing this book and knew I'd get there eventually but in my own time.

About the Author

The Author has always been someone who gets things done. Her mantras are 'no matter what', 'whatever it takes' and 'there's always a way'.

From being recognised in 2007 by Insider magazine as one of South Wales' "Top 20 Entrepreneurs to Watch" and finding herself sitting on the IOD Wales Management committee the author is all about shining brightly herself and supporting others out of the wings and into their spotlight so they too can shine brightly in their own production.

The author has had her fair share of hiding in the wings and when her industry leading business became insolvent overnight she was plunged into the turmoil of taking her own business through administration and personal bankruptcy. Her second marriage collapsed and she went through three redundancies. She suffered panic attacks, agoraphobia and more. For a while she thought she might stay in the wings forever but the lure of the spotlight proved too much of a draw.

The Author knew that she couldn't (and wouldn't) spend the rest of her life hiding in the wings, she decided she would get back into her spotlight no matter what and whatever it took.

She created a plan, a rehearsal schedule if you like, that enabled her to do just that. Deborah is passionate about enabling other people to create their own rehearsal schedule to move them gently out of the wings into their own spotlight.

The Author now lives the life she has always wanted. She has amazing relationships with the two most important people in her life; her partner and her son. She says, "I have regular holidays and I'm fitter and healthier than I've ever been."

As a coach she helps people move out of the wings into their spotlight so that they can become the star of their own life production. "And as far as I'm concerned, this is just the opening number."

Lightning Source UK Ltd.
Milton Keynes UK
UKHW02f2328020718

325137UK00008B/130/P